Acetylcholine - Recent Advances and New Perspectives

Edited by Thomas Heinbockel

Published in London, United Kingdom

Acetylcholine - Recent Advances and New Perspectives
http://dx.doi.org/10.5772/intechopen.106304
Edited by Thomas Heinbockel

Contributors
Vandana Mohan, Dhirender Kaushik, Komal Arora, Suresh Narayanan Nair, Presannan Usha Aswathy, Basavapura Mahadevappa Sanjay, Sanis Juliet, Mohit Vijay Vijay Rojekar, Kaushalraj Sunil Dandegonker, Swati Ghanghurde, Dongmei Ye, Susan Rempe, Lisa M. Savage, Matthew Fecik, Thomas Heinbockel, Yousef Tizabi, Bruk Getachew, Vassiliy Tsytsarev, Antonei B. Csoka, Robert L. L. Copeland

First published in London, United Kingdom, 2023 by IntechOpen
IntechOpen is the global imprint of INTECHOPEN LIMITED, registered in England and Wales, registration number: 11086078, 5 Princes Gate Court, London, SW7 2QJ, United Kingdom

British Library Cataloguing-in-Publication Data
A catalogue record for this book is available from the British Library

Additional hard and PDF copies can be obtained from orders@intechopen.com

Acetylcholine - Recent Advances and New Perspectives
Edited by Thomas Heinbockel
p. cm.
Print ISBN 978-1-80355-597-3
Online ISBN 978-1-80355-598-0
eBook (PDF) ISBN 978-1-80355-599-7

Meet the editor

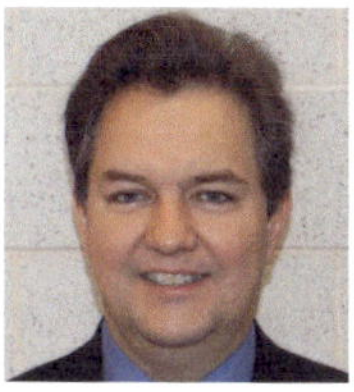

Thomas Heinbockel, Ph.D., is a professor in the Department of Anatomy, Howard University College of Medicine, Washington, DC, USA. He holds an adjunct faculty position in both the Department of Anatomy and Neurobiology and the Department of Physiology at University of Maryland School of Medicine. Dr. Heinbockel studied biology at Philipps University, Germany. His studies of the brain began during his MS thesis work at the Max-Planck-Institute for Behavioral Physiology, Germany. Dr. Heinbockel earned a Ph.D. in Neuroscience at the University of Arizona, USA. After graduating, he worked as a research associate at the Institute of Physiology, Otto-von-Guericke University, Germany. Dr. Heinbockel's research is focused on understanding how the brain processes information as it relates to neurological and psychiatric disorders. His laboratory at Howard University concentrates on foundational and translational topics such as drug development, organization of the olfactory and limbic systems, neural signaling, and synaptic transmission in the central nervous system.

Contents

Preface

This book, *Acetylcholine – Recent Advances and New Perspectives*, comes more than 100 years after the discovery of acetylcholine as a neurotransmitter in 1921 by Otto Loewi. Since then, the study of this neurotransmitter has been a magnificent chronicle in terms of its chemistry, biochemistry, function in the central and peripheral nervous system, and its relevance for neurological disorders and diseases. To this day, the study of acetylcholine and its receptors astounds us with novel features and exciting news. This book focuses on the role of this neurotransmitter in the physiology of individual neurons as well as in neural circuits and specific brain regions. It illustrates acetylcholine in all its dimensions, from historical perspectives to technological advances, as well as the use of novel tools in health and disease, in various animal models and organisms related to this critical neurotransmitter. Targeted at students and researchers in biological, chemical, medical and history disciplines, this book provides an overview of the work that is being done on this key signaling molecule of the nervous system and brain and highlights any gaps and areas that would benefit from further exploration.

The book is organized into two sections. Section 1, "Acetylcholine, Receptors and Diseases", includes five chapters. Section 2 "Acetylcholine Esterase, Neurotoxin", includes two chapters.

Chapter 1, "Introductory Chapter: The Neurotransmitter Acetylcholine – A Young Centenarian" by Thomas Heinbockel, outlines the events leading to the discovery of acetylcholine as a neurotransmitter and the role that Otto Loewi and Henry Dale played in its discovery.

In Chapter 2, "Avian Muscarinic Receptors: An Update", Presannan Usha Aswathy, Suresh Narayanan Nair, Basavapura Mahadevappa Sanjay and Sanis Juliet take the reader to the world of birds. The authors review the distribution of avian muscarinic receptor subtypes, the characterization of muscarinic acetylcholine receptors in various organs and organ systems, and the sequence similarity of muscarinic acetylcholine receptor subtypes between various birds and animals.

Chapter 3, "Central Nicotinic and Muscarinic Receptors in Health and Disease" by Yousef Tizabi, Bruk Getachew, Vassiliy Tsytsarev, Antonei B. Csoka, Robert L. Copeland and Thomas Heinbockel, provides a detailed account of the interaction of nicotinic and muscarinic acetylcholine receptors. Following a brief description of acetylcholine actions and its central circuitry, the authors give an update on muscarinic and nicotinic acetylcholine receptors and how their interaction may impact neuropsychiatric and neurodegenerative diseases. Finally, the authors touch upon potential novel therapeutic interventions based on these interactions, particularly in relation to Alzheimer and Parkinson disease.

Chapter 4, "Modes of Acetylcholine Signaling in the Prefrontal Cortex: Implications for Cholinergic Dysfunction and Disorders" by Matthew Fecik and Lisa M. Savage, reviews the current views on the functional role of phasic versus tonic cholinergic signaling, the contributions of acetylcholine receptors, hydrolysis, and basal forebrain anatomy. The authors also examine the implications of these factors in acetylcholine signaling in terms of cholinergic circuit dysfunction that occurs in neurodegenerative diseases.

In Chapter 5, "Role of Acetylcholine in Chronic Diseases", Vandana Mohan, Dhirender Kaushik and Komal Arora provide a brief overview of acetylcholine, including its synthesis and degradation, the cholinergic system, and the influence of acetylcholine on different chronic diseases, including neurological complications, metabolic disorders, cardiac diseases, and immune disorders. The authors review the mechanistic approach of acetylcholine in different diseases and the therapies for recovering the levels of acetylcholine.

In Chapter 6, "Paraoxonase in Nervous System", Mohit Vijay Rojekar, Kaushalraj Sunil Dandegonker and Swati Ghanghurde address the paraoxonase (PON) family, which consists of three enzymes that are anti-oxidative. Any dysfunction in their action can play a role in the pathobiology of diseases that have a chronic inflammatory component. Relevant to this book, the PON family interacts with acetylcholine esterase (AChE), and PONs degrade the inhibitors of AChE, which can affect the prognosis of the treatment of Alzheimer disease by inhibitors of organophosphates.

In Chapter 7, "Neurotoxin Decontamination", Dongmei Ye and Susan Rempe discuss how nerve agents, a group of organophosphorus (OP) compounds, are potent neurotoxins used as chemical warfare agents and insecticides. OP nerve agents disrupt the CNS by inhibiting AChE function. The authors discuss strategies to counter OP agents using organophosphorus hydrolase (OPH), a bacterial enzyme that can detoxify a wide range of OP agents. In their studies, the authors optimized OPH by incorporating selected unnatural amino acids into OPH, with mutations targeting both active and allosteric binding sites.

I am grateful to IntechOpen for initiating this book project and for asking me to serve as its editor. Many thanks go to Maja Bozicevic at IntechOpen for guiding me through the publication process and for moving the book ahead in a timely fashion. Thanks are due to all contributors to this book for taking the time to first write their chapter proposals, compose their chapters, and make the requested revisions. Hopefully, all contributors will continue their research with many intellectual challenges and exciting new directions. I would like to thank my wife Dr. Vonnie D.C. Shields, associate dean and professor, Towson University, MD, USA, and our son Torben Heinbockel for the time that I was able to spend working on this book project during the past year. Finally, I am grateful to my parents Erich and Renate Heinbockel for their continuous support and interest in my work over many years.

Thomas Heinbockel, Ph.D.
Department of Anatomy,
Howard University College of Medicine,
Washington, DC, USA

Section 1

Acetylcholine, Receptors and Diseases

Chapter 1

Introductory Chapter: The Neurotransmitter Acetylcholine – A Young Centenarian

Thomas Heinbockel

1. Introduction

If you are fortunate enough to grow in age and turn 100 years old, you are a centenarian. That is the term used for those human folks who are 100 years or older. The term is not typically applied to neurotransmitters. However, the neurotransmitter acetylcholine was discovered a little more than one hundred years ago, in 1921, by German-born scientist Otto Loewi. While human folks might face their final farewell at this age, current research on acetylcholine is testament to its young age, making it a young centenarian. As a PhD student in the Neuroscience program at the University of Arizona [https://neuroscience.arizona.edu/], my fellow students and I learned about acetylcholine as one of the major neurotransmitters in the nervous system, its synthesis, breakdown, and recycling [1, 2]. The fascinating story of acetylcholine's discovery and its functional importance for brain signaling upheld my continuous interest in this neurotransmitter.

2. Otto Loewi and his famous experiments

At the beginning of the 20th century, Loewi had worked on cardiac physiology for several years and published a continuous stream of papers in Pflügers Archiv (Pflüger's Archiv für die gesamte Physiologie des Menschen und der Tiere; today: Pflügers Archiv: European Journal of Physiology), the oldest physiological journal [3, 4]. The question that concerned scientists at the time was the mechanism that changed the beating frequency of the heart. Two alternatives presented themselves. In one of them, the heart itself released a substance that changed its beating frequency, whereas the other one postulated that some substance was released by nerve fibers, i.e., a form of chemical transmission existed [5]. In 1921, Loewi published a short paper [6] in this regard that described the key experiment carried out by him. It was a series of fortunate circumstances that led to his discovery of chemical transmission with acetylcholine as the messenger [7].

Loewi has recounted the nights before the critical experiment as he dreamt about it in his sleep [5]. The experiment used one frog heart where the vagus nerve was stimulated with electrical impulses. Electrical stimulation of the vagus nerve slowed down the heartbeat. The liquid from that heart (saline solution, i.e., Ringer's solution) was collected and applied to a second heart. The application resulted in a reduction in the beating frequency of the second heart. Loewi interpreted the slowing down of the second heart to mean that the vagus nerve had released a substance, the 'Vagusstoff' or vagus substance (acetylcholine) and proved that a soluble chemical released by the vagus nerve was controlling the heart rate. The chemical substance affected the heart rate through a process of chemical transmission [8]. The solution from the first heart slowed the second heart, and its beats diminished exactly as if its vagus nerve had been stimulated. In an additional experiment, Loewi stimulated the accelerator nerve of the first heart. When the nerve was stimulated and the Ringer solution from this heart was transferred, the second heart accelerated, and its beats increased [9]. Through these experiments, Loewi had solved the problem of determining whether any substance originated in the heart muscle to inhibit or activate it or whether the substance originated from the innervating nerve. In 1922, Loewi published a companion paper in which he ruled out the possibility that the chemical substances came from the heart [10]. In these experiments, he used high doses of nicotine which paralyzed the donor heart. Nevertheless, it was still possible to collect and transfer the Vagusstoff or the Acceleransstoff (adrenaline or epinephrine) from the paralyzed heart after stimulating the nerve. The idea for the initial experiment came to Loewi in a dream which prompted him to immediately go the lab after he woke up and carry out the experiment at 3 am in the morning [5, 11, 12]. His hypothesis of chemical transmission that he had postulated years earlier was proved by 5 am in the morning [11]. Loewi was lucky to carry out the experiment in a specific frog species at the time of day (diurnal cycle of the frog) and year that he did. The enzyme acetylcholinesterase rapidly metabolizes acetylcholine and could have prevented its effect on the heart. It was no surprise that chemical transmission was discovered in the peripheral nervous system as it affected visceral organs and skeletal muscles [5]. The experimental preparations were more accessible, and it was feasible to study drug effects. Moreover, chemical transmission was realized because certain drugs mimicked the stimulation of the autonomic nervous system that innervated visceral organs.

3. Henry Hallett Dale: friend and colleague

The other key player in the discovery of acetylcholine is Henry Hallett Dale who described acetylcholine as a neurochemical in 1914 [13]. In 1902 and subsequent years, Loewi visited the lab of Ernest Starling in London, England [12]. During those visits, he met Dale who, just like Loewi, was focused on biomedical bench work instead of clinical practice. Both became colleagues and lifelong friends. Dale's work included the isolation and identification of neurochemicals such as histamine and acetylcholine. He distinguished muscarinic and nicotinic acetylcholine activity which was instrumental for the later discovery of acetylcholine receptor classes and subtypes. Furthermore, based on the relatively transient effect of acetylcholine, Dale proposed the existence of an esterase that rapidly metabolized acetylcholine. Dale's findings laid the groundwork for Loewi's innovative discoveries. As a result of their cutting-edge and transformative research, 'the Nobel Prize in Physiology or Medicine 1936 was awarded jointly to Sir Henry Hallett Dale and Otto Loewi for their discoveries relating to chemical transmission of nerve impulses' [14]. Their work and discoveries were not without opposition in the field [15]. The famous neurophysiologist John Eccles believed that transmission at synapses was too fast to be carried out with chemicals. He thought that synaptic excitation had to be an electric process instead of a chemical one. The debate went on for several years in the middle of the 20th century. While Eccles initial idea was shown to be incorrect, he inadvertently helped Dale and others in the field to accomplish key experiments which proved chemical synaptic transmission in the peripheral and central nervous system. Eccles changed his opinion in the early 1950's after carrying out microelectrode experiments in his own lab. From then on, he was convinced of the existence of chemical synaptic transmission which he shared in a letter with Dale [5].

Acknowledgements

The author thanks the lab personnel for contributing to ongoing studies in his lab.

Funding

This publication resulted in part from research support to T.H. from the National Science Foundation [NSF IOS-1355034], Howard University College of Medicine, and the District of Columbia Center for AIDS Research, an NIH funded program [P30AI117970], which is supported by the following NIH Co-Funding and Participating Institutes and Centers: NIAID, NCI, NICHD, NHLBI, NIDA, NIMH, NIA, NIDDK, NIMHD, NIDCR, NINR, FIC and OAR. The content is solely the responsibility of the authors and does not necessarily represent the official views of the NIH.

Conflict of interest

The author declares that there is no conflict of interests regarding the publication of this chapter.

Author details

Thomas Heinbockel
Department of Anatomy, Howard University College of Medicine, Washington, DC, USA

*Address all correspondence to: theinbockel@howard.edu

References

[1] Nicholls JG, Martin AR, Wallace BG, Fuchs PA. From Neuron to Brain. 4th ed. Sunderland, MA: Sinauer Associates; 2001

[2] Kandel ER, Schwartz JH, Jessell TM. Principles of Neural Science. 4th ed. New York: McGraw-Hill; 2000

[3] Loewi O. Über die Beziehungen zwischen Herzmittel- und physiologischer Kationenwirkung. IV. Mitteilung. Über Nichtelektrolytwirkung aufs Herz. Pflügers Arch. 1921;**187**:105-122. DOI: 10.1007/BF01722069

[4] Loewi O. Über die Beziehungen zwischen Herzmittel- und physiologischer Kationenwirkung. IV. Mitteilung. Über die Wirkung von Lipoiden auf die Hypodynamie und deren Beziehung zum Kalium. Pflügers Archiv. 1921;**187**:123-131. DOI: 10.1007/BF01722070

[5] Valenstein ES. The discovery of chemical neurotransmitters. Brain and Cognition. 2002;**49**(1):73-95. DOI: 10.1006/brcg.2001.1487

[6] Loewi O. Über humorale übertragbarkeit der Herznervenwirkung. I. Mitteilung. Pflügers Arch. 1921;**189**:239-242. DOI: 10.1007/BF01738910

[7] Friedman AH. Circumstances influencing Otto Loewi's discovery of chemical transmission in the nervous system. Pflügers Archiv. 1971;**325**:85-86. DOI: 10.1007/BF00587494

[8] Borges R, García AG. One hundred years from Otto Loewi experiment, a dream that revolutionized our view of neurotransmission. Pflügers Arch-Eur J Physiol. 1921;**473**:977-981. DOI: 10.1007/s00424-021-02580-9

[9] Loewi O. An autobiographical sketch. Perspectives in Biology and Medicine. 1960;**4**:3-25

[10] Loewi O. Über humorale Übertragbarkeit der Herznervenwirkung. II. Mitteilung. Pflügers Archiv. 1922;**193**:201-213. DOI: 10.1007/BF02331588

[11] Loewi O. From the Workshop of Discoveries. Lawrence: Univ. of Kansas Press; 1953

[12] McCoy AN, Tan SY. Otto Loewi (1873-1961): Dreamer and Nobel laureate. Singapore Medical Journal. 2014;**55**(1):3-4. DOI: 10.11622/smedj.2014002

[13] Dale HH. The action of certain esters and ethers of choline, and their relation to muscarine. Journal of Pharmacology and Experimental Therapeutics. 1914;**6**(2):147-190

[14] The Nobel Prize in Physiology or Medicine 1936. NobelPrize.org. Nobel Prize Outreach AB 2023. Tue. 2023. Available from: https://www.nobelprize.org/prizes/medicine/1936/summary/

[15] Todman D. Henry Dale and the discovery of chemical synaptic transmission. European Neurology. 2008;**60**(3):162-164. DOI: 10.1159/000145336

Chapter 2

Avian Muscarinic Receptors: An Update

Presannan Usha Aswathy, Suresh Narayanan Nair, Basavapura Mahadevappa Sanjay and Sanis Juliet

Abstract

Muscarinic acetylcholine receptors (mAChRs) are widely expressed in both the central nervous system and peripheral nervous system and play a crucial role in modulating cellular activity and function. While these receptors have been extensively studied in mammals, their presence and role in avian species remain a relatively unexplored area of research. Nonetheless, several studies have suggested the existence of multiple functional muscarinic receptors in various avian species, including the vestibular periphery of pigeons, retinal cells, intestinal smooth muscles, dorsal root ganglia, developing hearts in chickens, and avian salt glands. Despite this, only the M2-M5 subtypes have been characterized, except for some studies that suggest the existence of functional M1 receptors in avian species, such as in the dorsal root ganglia, retina, heart, and vestibular periphery. In this paper, we review the distribution of avian muscarinic receptor subtypes, the characterization of muscarinic acetylcholine receptors in various organs and organ systems, and the sequence similarity of mAChR 2 and mAChR 3 between various birds and animals. Given the current gaps in our understanding, more research is needed to investigate further the function and expression of mAChRs in avian species.

Keywords: avian, muscarinic receptors, acetyl choline, birds, update, homology modeling, phylogeny tree, organs

1. Introduction

It is well established that mammals have got multiple functional receptors for neurotransmitters, and their role in the physiology of lower vertebrates is still less explored. Neurotransmitters are signal molecules with a confirmed neuronal release [1]. Among the different types of neurotransmitters, the major neurotransmitter released is acetylcholine (ACh) [2]. There are two types of acetylcholine receptors (AChRs) which are the nicotinic acetylcholine receptors (nAChRs) and the muscarinic acetylcholine receptors (mAChRs). Of these, the muscarinic receptors, are membrane proteins that belong to the superfamily of G-protein coupled receptors (GPCRs) that transmit their signals into the cell through heterotrimeric GTP-binding proteins (G-proteins), having seven transmembrane domains [3]. mAChRs are the most predominant cholinergic receptors in the central and peripheral nervous systems which plays an important role in modulating cell activity and function [4].

Moreover, muscarinic receptors are present in virtually all organs with a predominance of individual subtypes in various tissues and organs [5]. There are five genetically distinct subtypes of mammalian mAChRs (M1-M5) [6] in neurons and other cell types. M1, M4, and M5 receptors are most abundant in the central nervous system (CNS), while M2 and M3 receptors are widely distributed in both central and peripheral tissues [7]. The structural diversity between the five different mAChR subtypes is attributed to the presence of the residues in the third intracellular loop of the protein [8]. Experiments like Northern blot and *in situ* hybridization have revealed that there is some tissue specificity in the distribution of receptor subtype mRNAs. Muscarinic subtypes have also been distinguished based on tissue-specific antagonists and have been developed for therapeutic purposes [5].

The M1 mAChR subtype is abundant in the brain and enteric nervous system while the M2 mAChR subtype is mainly expressed in the heart. Peripheral M3 mAChRs are found extensively in smooth muscles of the gastrointestinal and urinary tracts, exocrine glands, and the eye [9]. In the periphery, M4 mAChRs have been found in relatively higher concentrations in the lungs and in lower concentrations in the salivary glands and ileum. Various peripheral and cerebral blood vessels have been used for the study and identification of mRNA for M5 mAChRs [7]. The M1, M3, and M5 subtypes are tightly coupled to the phosphoinositide system, whereas the M2 and M4 subtypes are closely linked to the mechanism of adenylate cyclase inhibition [10].

Many biochemical and histochemical studies have illustrated evolutionary changes in terms of the concentration of acetylcholine in different parts of the brains of the lower vertebrates [11]. Another study [12] has proposed an increasing functional role for acetylcholine in some telencephalic structures, particularly in the basal ganglia and the tuberculum olfactorium in lower vertebrates. The basal ganglia in non-mammalian brains are extremely enriched in AChE (acetylcholine esterase) activity like that in mammals, while differences in the concentration and distribution of this enzyme occur in the cerebellum of the vertebrate brain [13]. Some studies report chicken may have a cholinergic habenulointerpeduncular pathway system identical to that reported in the rat [14] which suggests the existence of cholinergic cell bodies and fibers in the avian brain. The study has confirmed the above results using immunohistochemical localization of choline acetyltransferase in the chicken mesencephalon, which is part of the avian midbrain.

However, despite the characterization and cloning of all muscarinic receptor subtypes in different species, to date, there are no reports of a functional M1 muscarinic receptor in chicken. This article focuses on the avian muscarinic receptors, their subtypes, distribution, expression as well as characterization and reviews the available information about the various research held in this field so far.

2. Structure of avian muscarinic receptors using homology modeling

So far, there are no reported structures for avian muscarinic receptors in protein data bank or any other public domain sites. We used homology modeling to build the receptor structure using protein-BLAST search (Sequence ID for this search are provided with the individual structures - see **Figure 1**). Homology modeling is used to determine three-dimensional structure of proteins using its amino acid sequence. It is a model used for computational structure prediction of proteins. Afterwards the SWISS-MODEL service (https://swissmodel.expasy.org/) was used to model the tertiary structure using suggested template protein structure. Discovery Studio Client was

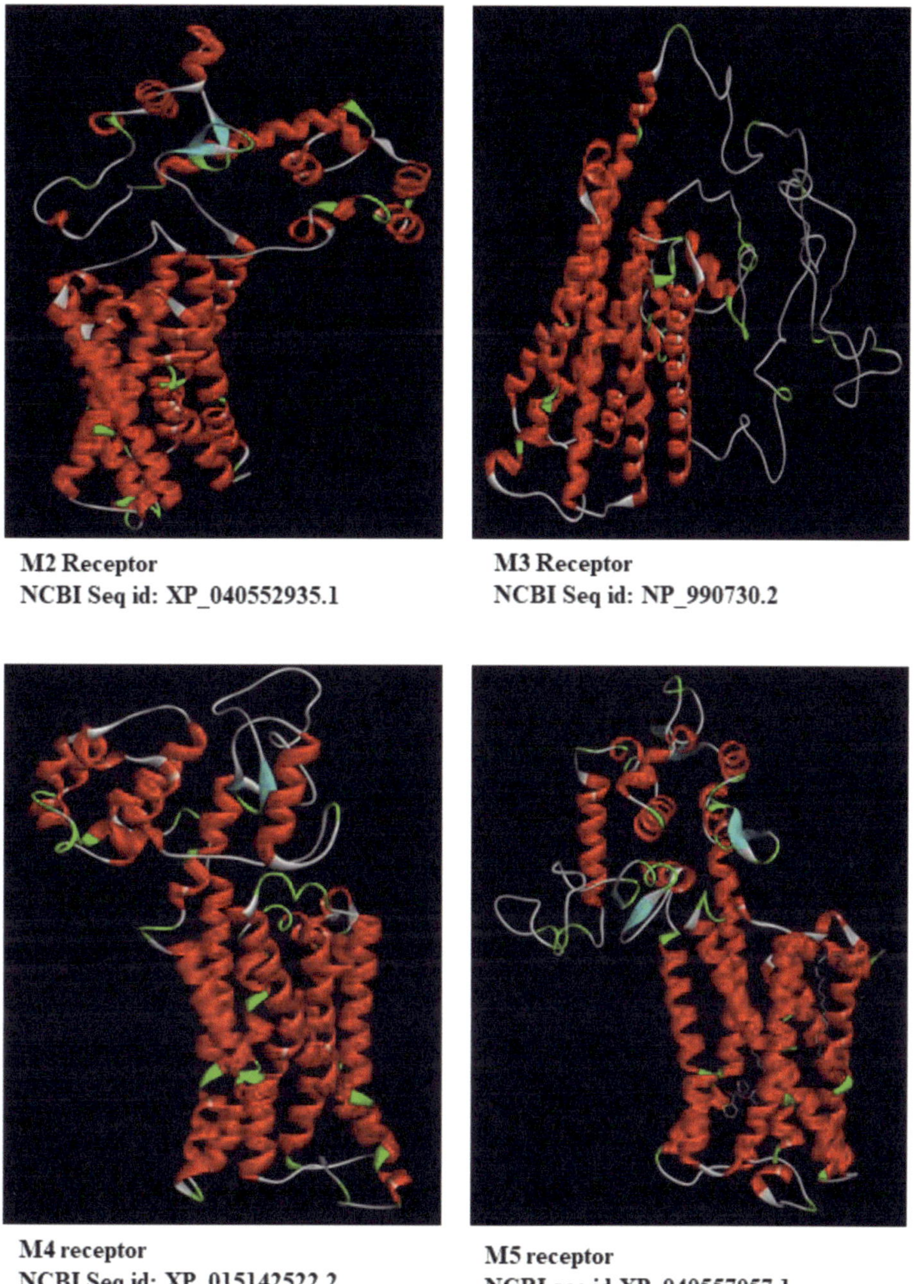

Figure 1.
Images of muscarinic acetylcholine receptor subtypes reported in chicken (Gallus gallus domesticus) homology modeled using Swiss model (https://swissmodel.expasy.org/).

used to visualize the final model (**Figure 1**). In the picture the visual similarities and differences between M2, M3, M4, and M5 are visible. By doing nucleotide sequence alignment, it has been shown that there are not many similarities between each of the muscarinic receptors, though acetylcholine can bind with all the receptors. This may be due to the similar sequences in the ligand binding domains of all the four receptors.

3. Comparison of sequences and construction of phylogenic tree of avian muscarinic subsets

Multiple sequence alignment was done with NCBI tool (https://www.ncbi.nlm.nih.gov/blast/) and individual phylogenic tree for each receptor among avian were created using MEGA 11. Respective human receptors were used for comparative purpose (**Figures 2–4**) similarity between the reported avian sequences as shown in

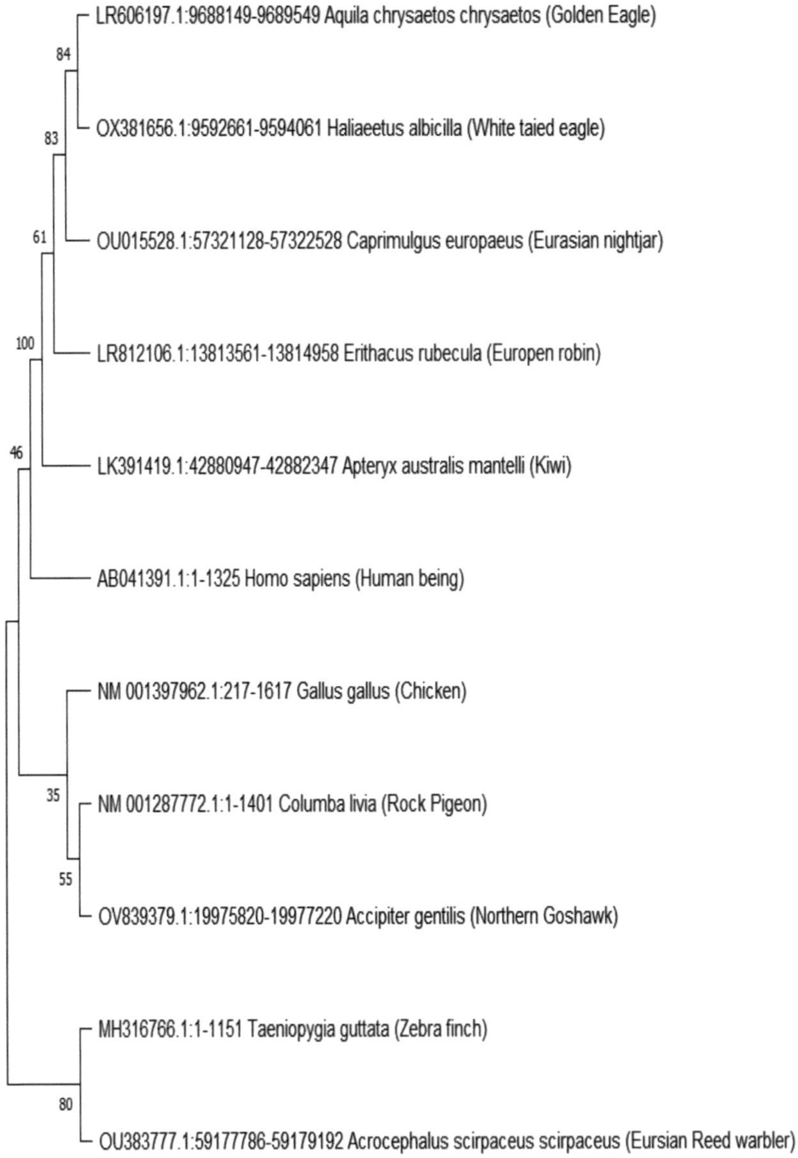

Figure 2.
Phylogeny tree prepared based on sequence similarity of mAChR 2 of C. livia with different species prepared using MEGA11.

the tables (**Tables 1–3**). By analyzing **Table 1** the percentage identity of mAChR 2 of *Columba livia* (rock pigeon) with that of *Aquila chrysaetos* (golden eagle) is 95.5% with maximum percentage similarity and minimum similarity with cholinergic muscarinic receptor 2 of *Homo sapiens* (human beings). Similarly, **Table 3** details gives percentage identity of muscarinic receptor 3 with other species and its respective human receptors. The same applies to **Table 4** and **Figure 4**.

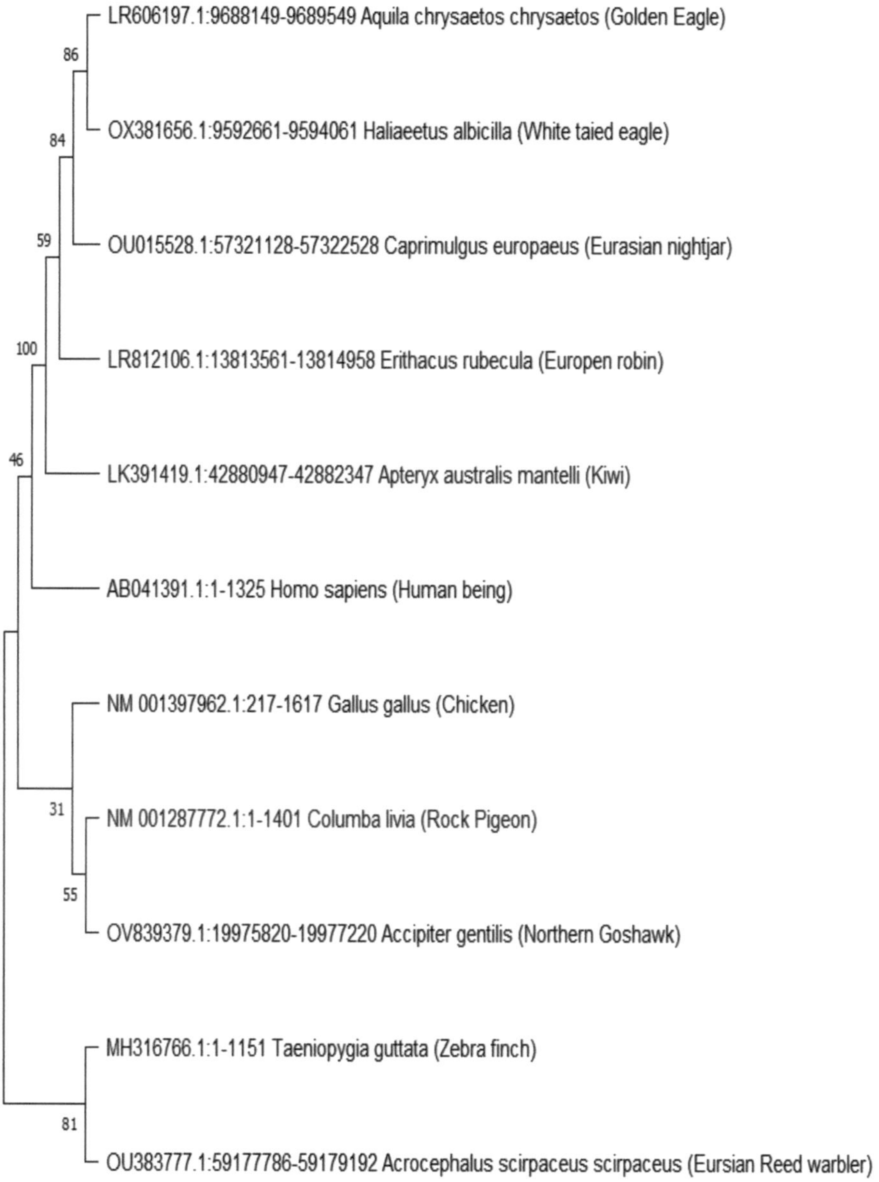

Figure 3.
Phylogeny tree prepared based on sequence similarity of mAChR 3 of C. livia with different species prepared using MEGA.

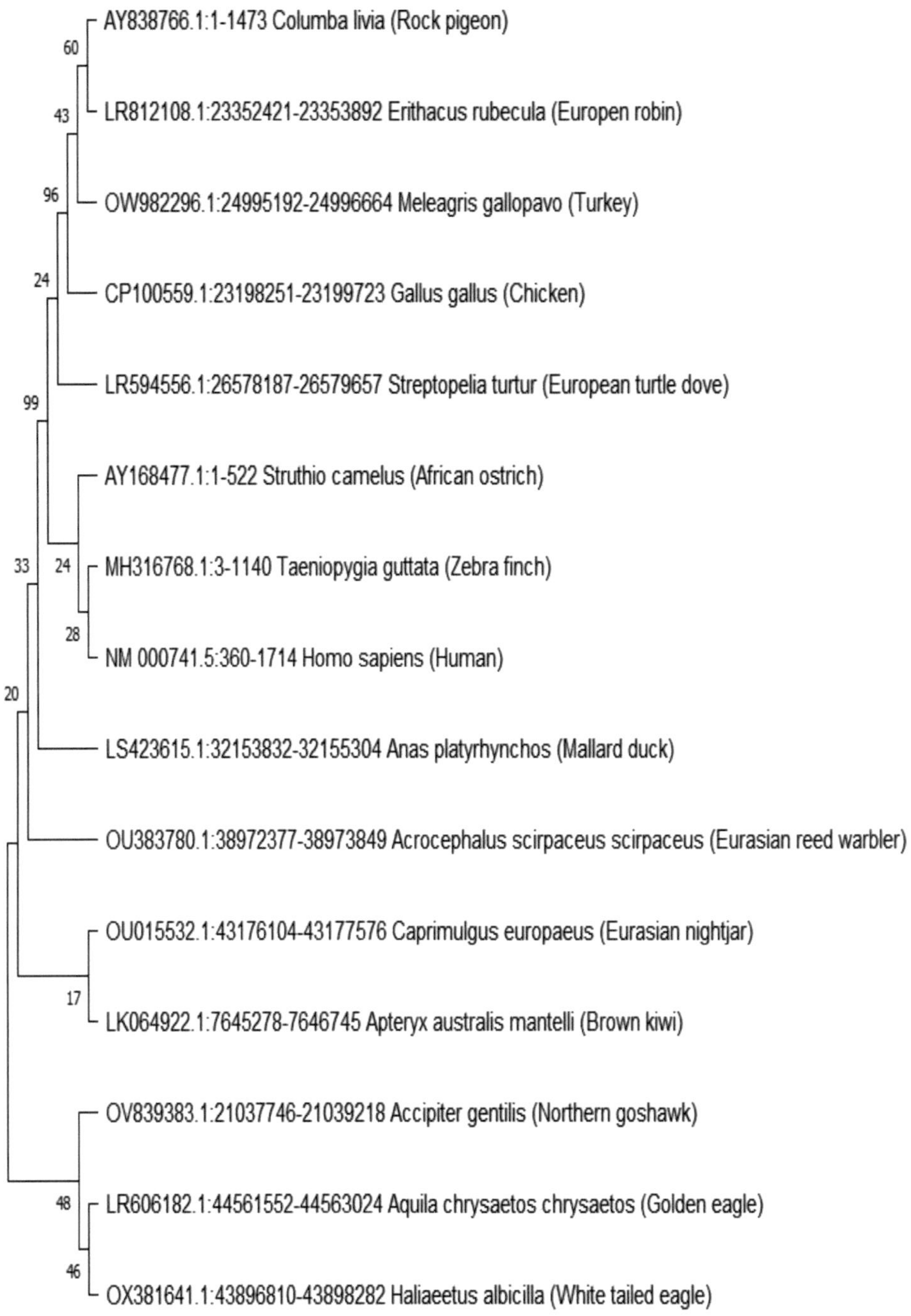

Figure 4.
Phylogeny tree prepared based on sequence similarity of mAChR 4 of C.livia with different species prepared using MEGA11.

Sl No	Description	Scientific Name and Common Name	Percent identity	Accession
1	*C. livia* cholinergic receptor muscarinic 2 (CHRM2), mRNA	*C. livia* (rock pigeon)	100	NM_001287772.1
2	*Aquila chrysaetos chrysaetos* genome assembly, chromosome: 17	*A. chrysaetos chrysaetos* (Golden Eagle)	95.5	LR606197.1
3	*Haliaeetus albicilla* genome assembly, chromosome: 19	*H. albicilla* (White-tailed eagle)	95.36	OX381656.1
4	*Accipiter gentilis* genome assembly, chromosome: 18	*A. gentilis* (Northern goshawk)	95.36	OV839379.1
5	*Caprimulgus europaeus* genome assembly, chromosome: 5	*C. europaeus* (Eurasian nightjar)	94.86	OU015528.1
6	*Apteryx australis mantelli* genome assembly AptMant0, scaffold scaffold27	*Apteryx mantelli* (Kiwi)	92.93	LK391419.1
7	*Gallus gallus* cholinergic receptor muscarinic 2 (CHRM2), transcript variant 2, mRNA	*G. gallus* (chicken)	91.86	NM_001397962.1
8	*Acrocephalus scirpaceus scirpaceus* genome assembly, chromosome: 4	*A. scirpaceus scirpaceus* (Reed Warbler)	91.13	OU383777.1
9	*Erithacus rubecula* genome assembly, chromosome: 4	*E. rubecula* (European robin)	91.08	LR812106.1
10	*Taeniopygia guttata* muscarinic acetylcholine receptor 2 (chrm2) mRNA, partial cds	*T. guttata* (zebra finch)	91.51	MH316766.1
11	*H. sapiens* cholinergic receptor muscarinic 2 (CHRM2), transcript variant 5, mRNA	*H. sapiens* (human)	79.15	NM_001006631.3

Table 1.
Sequence similarity of mAChR 2 of C. livia with different species. Data collected from pubmed (https://www.ncbi.nlm.nih.gov/) and created with NCBI-nucleotide-BLAST (https://www.ncbi.nlm.nih.gov/blast/).

Sl No.	Description	Scientific Name and Common Name	Per. ident	Accession
1	*C. livia* cholinergic receptor muscarinic 3 (CHRM3), mRNA	*C. livia* (Rock pigeon)	100	NM_001282818.1
2	*Haliaeetus albicilla* genome assembly, chromosome: 13	*H. albicilla* (White-tailed eagle)	96.27	OX381650.1
3	*Accipiter gentilis* genome assembly, chromosome: 28	*A. gentilis* (Northern goshawk)	96.11	OV839389.1
4	*A. chrysaetos* chrysaetos genome assembly, chromosome: 13	*A. chrysaetos* (Golden Eagle)	95.89	LR606193.1

Sl No.	Description	Scientific Name and Common Name	Per. ident	Accession
5	*Gallus gallus* cholinergic receptor muscarinic 3 (CHRM3), transcript variant 1, mRNA	*G. gallus* (Chicken)	93.23	NM_205399.2
6	*Apteryx australis mantelli* genome assembly AptMant0, scaffold scaffold19	*Apteryx mantelli* (Brown kiwi)	93.28	LK064669.1
7	*Taeniopygia guttata* muscarinic acetylcholine receptor 3 (chrm3) mRNA, partial cds	*T. guttata* (zebra finch)	93.93	MH316767.1
8	*Corvus splendens* muscarinic acetylcholine receptor M3 mRNA, partial cds	*C. splendens* (House crow)	95.01	MW036511.1
9	*H. sapiens* cholinergic receptor muscarinic 3 (CHRM3), transcript variant 10, mRNA	*H. sapiens* (Human)	79.11	NM_001375985.1

Table 2.
Sequence similarity of mAChR 3 of C. livia with different species. Data collected from pubmed (https://www.ncbi.nlm.nih.gov/) and created with NCBI-nucleotide-BLAST (https://www.ncbi.nlm.nih.gov/blast/).

Sl No.	Description	Scientific Name and Common Name	Per. ident	Accession
1	*C. livia* brain acetylcholine muscarinic receptor sub-type 4 (Chrm4) mRNA, complete cds	*C. livia* (rock pigeon)	100	AY838766.1
2	*Streptopelia turtur* genome assembly, chromosome: 5	*S. turtur* (European Turtle Dove)	98.51	LR594556.1
3	*Caprimulgus europaeus* genome assembly, chromosome: 9	*C. europaeus* (Eurasian nightjar)	93.55	OU015532.1
4	*A. chrysaetos chrysaetos* genome assembly, chromosome: 2	*A. chrysaetos* (Golden Eagle)	93.41	LR606182.1
5	*Haliaeetus albicilla* genome assembly, chromosome: 5	*H. albicilla* (white-tailed eagle)	93.41	OX381641.1
6	*Accipiter gentilis* genome assembly, chromosome: 22	*A. gentilis* (Northern goshawk)	93.41	OV839383.1
7	*Apteryx australis mantelli* genome assembly AptMant0, scaffold scaffold87	*Apteryx mantelli* (Brown Kiwi)	92.57	LK064922.1
8	*Acrocephalus scirpaceus scirpaceus* genome assembly, chromosome: 7	*Acrocephalus scirpaceus* (Eurasian Reed Warbler)	92.26	OU383780.1
9	*Erithacus rubecula* genome assembly, chromosome: 6	*E. rubecula* (European robin)	91.99	LR812108.1
10	*Gallus gallus* breed Huxu chromosome 5	*G. gallus* (chicken)	91.85	CP100559.1
11	*Meleagris gallopavo* genome assembly, chromosome: 5	*M. gallopavo* (turkey)	91.65	OW982296.1

Sl No.	Description	Scientific Name and Common Name	Per. ident	Accession
12	*Anas platyrhynchos* genome assembly, chromosome: 5	*A. platyrhynchos* (mallard duck)	91.58	LS423615.1
13	*Taeniopygia guttata* muscarinic acetylcholine receptor 4 (chrm4) mRNA, partial cds	*T. guttata* (zebra finch)	92.83	MH316768.1
14	*H. sapiens* cholinergic receptor muscarinic 4 (CHRM4), transcript variant 1, mRNA	*H. sapiens* (human)	76.45	NM_000741.5
15	*Struthio camelus* acetylcholinergic receptor M4 (acm4) gene, partial cds	*S. camelus* (African ostrich)	91.57	AY168477.1

Table 3.
Sequence similarity of mAChR 4 of C. livia with different species. Data collected from pubmed (https://www.ncbi.nlm.nih.gov/) and created with NCBI-nucleotide-BLAST (https://www.ncbi.nlm.nih.gov/blast/).

Sl No.	Avian Species	Organ	Muscarinic Subtype	References
1	Herring gulls	Salt glands	Nonselective mAChR	Hootman and Ernst [15]
2	Chick	Lateral spiriform nucleus of CNS	M3	Guo and Chiappinelli [16]
3	Chick	Dorsal Root Ganglion (DRG)	M1, M3	Tata *et al.* [17]
4	Chicken	Dorsal Root Ganglion (DRG)	M1	Peralta *et al.* [3]
5	Chicken	Basilar artery in brain	M3	Matsumoto *et al.* [18]
6	Chicken	Heart (Atria)	M1	Jeck *et al.* [19]
7	Chicken (Broiler)	CNS	M1, M3	Zendehdel *et al.* [20]
8	Chick	Heart	M2	Tietje and Nathanson [14]
9	Chicken	Heart	M1	Brehm *et al.* [21]
10	Chick	Ventricle of heart	M1, M4	Nouchi *et al.* [22]
11	Chick	Brain, atria and ventricle	M3	Gadbut and Galper [23]
12	Chick	Heart and brain	M5	Creason *et al.* [24]
13	Chick	Ocular tissue	M2	Yin *et al.* [25]
14	Chick	Vitreous chamber of eye	M4	McBrien *et al.* [26]
15	Chicken	Proventriculus	M3	Kitazawa *et al.* [27]
16	Chicken	Ileum	M2, M3	Darroch *et al.* [28]
17	Chick	Choroid	M3	Fischer *et al.* [29] and Zagvazdin *et al.* [30]
18	Chicken	Trachea	M4	Winding and Bindslev [31]

Sl No.	Avian Species	Organ	Muscarinic Subtype	References
19	Pigeon	Vestibular end organs	M1, M2, M3, M4, M5	Li and Correia [32]
20	Quail	Rectum	Nonselective mAChR	Shiina and Takewaki [33]
21	Quail	Ileum	M2, M3	Sanjay *et al.* [34]

Table 4.
Distribution of subtypes of muscarinic receptors in various species and their location.

4. Location of avian muscarinic receptors

In birds, fundamental pharmacological studies indicate that mAChRs located in the CNS are associated with vision, navigation, metabolism, and central thermoregulation [35]. However, the role of each of the mAChRs subtypes has not been established in either the CNS or peripheral nervous system [36]. Muscarinic receptor subtypes are expressed in cochlear neurons, supporting cells, central auditory neurons [37], avian vestibular hair cells, nerve terminals, ganglion cells, [38] and also in the avian retina [39]. **Table 4** narrates the important locations of muscarinic receptors in birds.

4.1 Avian muscarinic receptors in the central nervous system

Even though the information on muscarinic receptor subtype M1 present in avians is few, some studies have given proof for the presence of central muscarinic M1 receptor subtype. A study [20] has reported the role of muscarinic receptor subtypes M1 and M3 involved in carbachol-induced hypophagia in neonatal broiler chicken. Moreover, the study provided first evidence for muscarinic receptor mediated hypophagic effect in domestic fowl and that the hypophagic effect of muscarinergic system is mediated via M1 and M3 receptors, which were similar to previous reports in mammals [40, 41]. In this study, M2 and M4 receptors had no role in feeding behavior in neonatal broiler chicken, but both M2 and M4 receptors had a prominent role in feeding behavior in rat [42]. It is a well-known fact that there is a significant difference on the role of neurotransmitters in the feeding behavior between avian and mammals [20].

Another study [16] was conducted to assess the functional role of muscarinic acetylcholine receptors in chick brain slices using whole-cell patch-clamp recordings of neurons in the lateral spiriform nucleus. The lateral spiriform nucleus (SpL) forms part of the avian basal ganglia system. It receives cholinergic innervation from the nucleus semilunaris, as well as glutamatergic input from the ansa lenticularis subthalamus, GABAergic input from the paleostriatum primitivum and both GABAergic and possibly dopaminergic inputs from the substantia nigra [43]. But their functional roles in influencing motor behavior remain largely unknown, even after depicting the anatomical pathways. Possibly, the ACh released from cholinergic nerve terminals in or close to the SpL enhances the release of GABA by means of nicotinic AChR activation, which is located on GABAergic axon terminals [44]. Similarly, ACh might act simultaneously on muscarinic AChRs also.

Results of their study revealed that bath application of carbachol, a muscarinic agonist, enhanced the frequency of spontaneous postsynaptic currents and produced a pronounced postsynaptic inward current in normal ACSF (Artificial Cerebrospinal Fluid) with a slower onset but more prolonged action. These effects may be due to the possible muscarinic AChRs belonging to the M3 subtype category and are located some distance from release sites, requiring activation of voltage-dependent sodium channels and N-type voltage-dependent calcium channels (VDCCs) to trigger enhanced GABA release. To determine the muscarinic receptor subtype that mediated enhancement of spontaneous GABAergic IPSCs (Inhibitory Postsynaptic Currents), several muscarinic antagonists were used for testing, of which 4- DAMP mustard alone completely blocked muscarine's effect. As per existing data on 4-DAMP mustard, it exhibits a high affinity for the M3 receptor, whereas its affinity for other subtypes is significantly lower [45]. Moreover, the pharmacological profile suggested that M3 receptors predominantly contributed to the muscarinic enhancement of GABA release, thus giving evidence for the same.

Another study reported a cDNA that encodes a chicken protein that is homologous to mammalian prion protein (PrPc). PrPc in mammals is an altered isoform of the infectious particle prion (PrP^{sc}) thought to be responsible for spongiform encephalopathies in humans and animals. It is a cellular protein of unknown function in mammals. Chicken prion-like protein (ch-PrLP) is expressed in embryos as early as day 6 in the central nervous system, mostly in the motor neurons. It was found that this protein is abundant in preparations of an acetylcholine receptor-inducing activity based on its ability to synthesize nicotinic receptors in cultured myotubes. Hence, according to the study, it is likely that they serve normally in the neuromuscular junction and central nervous system to regulate chemoreceptor numbers [46].

4.1.1 Muscarinic receptors in pigeon brain

The avian nidopallium caudolaterale (NCL), situated in the caudal telencephalon, serves comparable functions to the mammalian prefrontal cortex, although both are not homologous structures. In the last decades, assumed homologies between avian and mammalian brain components has been studied [47]. It assumes that mammalian and avian pallia share a homologous pallial identity that may be derived from a common ancestry [48]. However, this does not imply that cortical or subcortical pallial areas must be exactly homologous to pallial components in birds.

Various researchers have proved that the mammalian prefrontal cortex (PFC) and the avian NCL share several anatomical neurochemicals [49], electrophysiological and functional [50] characteristics. Hence, the similarities between NCL and PFC may likely do not result from common ancestry, but may be due to an evolutionary convergence. In a quantitative analysis of different receptor binding sites, using autoradiography, by labelling the muscarinic cholinergic M1 receptor with pirenzepine and the muscarinic cholinergic M2 receptor with oxotremorine, the study compared the receptor fingerprints of NCL with those of frontal areas in mammals.

ACh is an essential regulator of cortical excitability and plays important roles for arousal, attention, and cognitive processes [51, 52]. These functions are mediated by muscarinic and nicotinic ACh receptors. Cholinergic M1 receptors were highest in humans if compared to macaque monkey, rhesus monkey, rat and pigeon, while M2 and nicotinic receptors showed equal densities [53]. However, pigeons showed an inverted pattern of M1/M2 binding in the NCL compared to other species which suggests an increased inhibitory control on local circuits, this may be a compensating mechanism for the shift to glutamatergic processing which was at highest concentration in the avian nidopallium [54].

4.1.2 Muscarinic receptors in avian nerve fibers

DRG (dorsal root ganglia) is a collection of bipolar cell bodies of neurons, formed when the dorsal sensory root of spinal nerves exits the neural foramina, surrounded by layers of satellite glial cells (SGCs) [55]. DRG neurons are pseudo-unipolar cells. They give rise to one fiber from which both central and peripheral projections derive, forming peripheral and central sensory branches. These branches contain both myelinated and unmyelinated fibers differing in size, conduction velocity, and perception specification, e. g. nociceptive and thermal sensory neurons [56].

Immunocytochemical studies conducted in the chick DRGs has shown that muscarinic receptors are present in almost all neurons of DRG with a K_d value for [^{3}H]QNB (H-3-quinuclidinyl benzilate) comparable to that reported for mAChRs in other tissue with cholinergic innervation. Hence, DRG neurons not only express cholinergic neurotransmission markers, a high-affinity choline uptake system (HACU) [57], but are also muscarinic cholinoceptive [58]. Functional studies using d-tubocurarine in chick dorsal root ganglia have shown that only about 50% of DRG neurons are responsive to acetylcholine and are sensitive to dtubocurarine suggesting their nicotinic nature [59]. Thus, the divergent distribution of both muscarinic and nicotinic acetylcholine receptor types may indicate their different role in DRG neurons.

A similar study has also identified the presence of muscarinic cholinergic receptors and their microanatomical localization in chicken dorsal root ganglia. They used pirenzepine in competition binding experiments, which showed high affinity for the cloned M1 receptor and labels the M1 receptor of the pharmacological classification [3]. Though the absolute specificity of pirenzepine was questioned by many studies for M1 muscarinic cholinergic receptors [60], the sensitivity of [^{3}H]QNB binding to the compound suggests the expression of the M1 receptor subtype in chick DRG.

In another study to establish muscarinic receptors modulate intracellular calcium levels in sensory neurons of chicks, E18 embryonic chicks were treated with muscarinic agonists such as muscarine and oxotremorine which resulted in an increase of intracellular calcium levels in fura-2 AM (fluorescent calcium indicator) loaded DRG neurons. This effect was antagonized by treatment with atropine and not with the same concentration of mecamylamine indicating that the increase in calcium concentration was due to muscarinic receptor activation. To substantiate the above findings, selective antagonists of muscarinic receptor subtypes were tested, and it also indicated that M1 to a greater extent and to a lesser extent M3 receptor subtypes were responsible for the observed intracellular calcium mobilization. These findings suggest a functional role for acetylcholine and muscarinic receptors in sensory transduction [17]. Moreover, second messengers such as cGMP and cAMPs muscarinic modulation have already been reported in DRG neurons by demonstrating the presence of M1 and possibly M3 subtype in the chick dorsal root ganglia [58].

Another study conducted to investigate the presence of mAChRs by immunolabeling neurons, nerve fibers, Schwann cells, and satellite cells in chicken also suggests the presence of mAChR subtypes. It showed a consistent presence of mAChRs in the neuronal plasma membrane, which suggests a probable role for mAChRs during neuronal differentiation ad exchange of information between neurons [61]. In the nerve fibers, mAChR was detected in the initial segment of emerging neuronal fibers at E12, but the unmyelinated axons of both peripheral and central branches were devoid of an immunoreaction product. This indicates mAChRs may not be involved in the transduction of sensory stimuli [62] in early life. Later, in young chicks several unmyelinated fibers, both central and peripheral, become immunopositive. In young chicks, the immunoreaction product was detected in the axoplasm of numerous unmyelinated central axons, suggesting transport of mAChRs towards the nerve endings in the spinal cord.

In the satellite and Schwann cells, at E12 numerous perineuronal satellite cells surrounding the soma of immunopositive and immunonegative neurons were strongly labeled for mAChRs. Reciprocal communication between neurons and glial cells is well established [63]. Various neuroactive substances synthesized and released by glial cells are involved in neuronal differentiation and growth. Similarly, interaction between Schwann cells and axons are also important for the maintenance of structural integrity and functioning of axons. All these suggest a correlation that at early developmental stages of the avian DRG, the mAChRs expressed by satellite and Schwann cells is important to control the morphogenesis of neurons that take part in sensory functions as well as their axons.

4.1.3 Muscarinic receptors in avian Edinger-Westphal nucleus

Choroid in birds is extensively innervated by ciliary ganglion [64]. Edinger-Westphal (EW) nucleus is the source of the parasympathetic preganglionic input to the ciliary ganglion, upon electrical stimulation, increases the choroidal blood flow in pigeons [65]. Various pharmacological investigations suggest that NO (Nitric Oxide) mediates the EW-evoked vasodilatory response [66]. Earlier studies have identified M3 receptors in avian choroid [29], which mediates the tone of vascular beds in the avian choroid probably by the cholinergic-dependent release of endothelium-derived relaxing factor (presumably NO) [67, 68].

The study examined the role and the type of muscarinic receptors within the choroid that is involved in the increases in choroidal blood flow, using electrical stimulation of the nucleus of Edinger-Westphal (EW) nucleus to activate the ciliary ganglion input to choroid in pigeons. M3 receptors were blocked using a selective antagonist, 4-diphenyl-acetoxy-N-methylpiperedine (4-DAMP), it reduced the baseline choroidal blood flow. Simultaneously, atropine, a non-selective antagonist of muscarinic receptors, decreased the EW-evoked responses to a lesser extent than 4-DAMP.

The results of the study suggested a major role of M3 type muscarinic receptors in the EW evoked increases in choroidal blood flow in pigeons [30]. Based on another finding that the input of ciliary ganglion to choroid does not synthesize NO, but inhibitors of NO production do block EW-evoked choroidal vasodilation [66], it seems likely that the M3 receptors acted on by 4-DAMP are present on choroidal endothelial cells and mediate choroidal vasodilation via stimulation of endothelial release of nitric oxide.

5. Avian muscarinic receptors in sensory structures

5.1 Muscarinic receptors in avian vestibular end organs

Muscarinic acetylcholine receptor subtype expression in avian vestibular hair cells, nerve terminals and ganglion cells has been conducted based on the patch clamp recordings from pigeon native hair cells with carbachol, a cholinergic agonist, resulted in reduction of the current through the inward rectifier pKir2.1 channel [32]. The cilia on the hair cells and the associated structures are important during sensory transduction.

They cloned and sequenced pigeon mAChR subtypes M2–M5 in the pigeon vestibular end organs (semicircular canal ampullary cristae and utricular maculae), vestibular nerve fibers and the vestibular (Scarpa's) ganglion and studied the expression of all five mAChR subtypes (M1–M5) in the pigeon vestibular end organs (semicircular canal ampullary cristae and utricular maculae), vestibular using tissue immunohistochemistry (IH), dissociated single cell immunocytochemistry (IC) and Western blotting (WB). In the study, vestibular hair cells, nerve fibers and ganglion cells expressed all five (M1–M5) mAChR subtypes. mAChRs M1 and M5 were found on the nerve terminals, supporting cells, and cilia of hair cells. And mAChRs M1, M3 and M5 were expressed on cuticular plates, myelin sheaths and Schwann cells. M2 and M4 mAChRs were seen on the nerve terminals. M2 was also present on the cuticular plates and supporting cells [38].

Immunohistochemistry and Immunocytochemistry results were consistent with results from WB of the dissociated vestibular epithelia, nerve fibers and vestibular ganglia. It is clear from the study that the neuronal components of the labyrinth exhibit significant co-expression of the subtypes. Even though the study does not give data on quantitative expression of M1–M5 but do indicate that the mAChRs are widely present and co-expressed on elements in the vestibular peripheral system. The additional possibility of mAChR expression on efferent fibers and terminals forming autoreceptors should be analyzed using further research in this area.

Acetylcholine receptors often perform autocrine and neuronal activities [69]. Control of cell growth and proliferation and release of chemical mediators [70, 71] are the major autocrine functions. These functions are important in vestibular hair cell regeneration or maintenance and replenishment of endolymph and perilymph. Non-neuronal cholinergic function is attributed by the expression of mAChR subtypes on the supporting cells and Schwann cells [72].

5.2 Muscarinic receptors involved in chick myopia

Various studies conducted in the chick model of myopia has proved that the most effective anti-muscarinic agents for myopia includes the non-selective agents like atropine [73] and oxyphenonium [74], followed by the partially selective muscarinic antagonists M1 and M4 selective pirenzepine [75] and the M2 and M4 selective himbacine [76]. In a study using the selective M4 muscarinic receptor antagonist MT-3, it was effective in inhibiting form-deprivation myopia in the chick by means of inhibition of vitreous chamber elongation, the major structural cause of myopia, associated with inhibition of choroidal thinning in myopic chicks. While in certain studies using muscarinic antagonists such as atropine and pirenzepine, they also produced similar efficacy in reducing myopia, at doses substantially higher than that would be considered necessary for a muscarinic receptor-based mechanism, namely at micromolar concentrations.

But in this particular study, since the muscarinic antagonists applied were highly selective for the M4 and M1 receptors, the doses were calculated to be at nanomolar concentrations at the receptor level. Similarly, upon applying the highly selective M1 muscarinic antagonist MT-7, it had no inhibitory effect on form-deprivation myopia in chick, deriving a conclusion that the chick lacks an M1 receptor, as supported by their findings [26].

In a similar experiment involving the chick myopia model, attempts were made to isolate and process RNA and genomic DNA for the evidence of a functional M1 muscarinic receptor in chicken. However, the results produced no evidence for the same, which itself indicates that the mRNA template necessary for the production of the M1 receptor protein is unlikely to be present in chick. Furthermore, it could be concluded that the chick lacks a gene or promoter sequence for the M1 receptor. Moreover, the study was consistent with previous report, which demonstrates a tenfold affinity of pirenzepine for the chick M2 receptor subtype than its mammalian counterpart [77]. Hence, the study suggests the possibility that pirenzepine inhibits myopia progression via the M2 receptor in birds and via the M1 receptor in mammals. Furthermore, it also suggests the possibility that muscarinic antagonists which prevents myopia in chicks mediates its action through another muscarinic subtype, probably the M4 subtype or through non-specific or non-receptor mediated mechanisms [25].

Moreover, this can be consistent with another finding which localized the presence of G protein-coupled receptor kinases (GRKs) in the avian retina [39]. GRKs are enzymes that are involved in the phosphorylation of serine/threonine residues in the carboxy-terminal of various of agonist-occupied G protein-coupled receptors [78, 79]. Retinal morphology and electrophysiology are relatively well characterized, since it is an excellent model for neurochemical studies of the nervous system since its development. At least six enzymes have been cloned and were extensively characterized from mammals [80]. Of these, mammalian retinal rods and cones expressed GRK1 [81]. In the chicken retina, two different types of photoreceptors expressed a novel GRK1 [82]. However, not only muscarinic receptors act via GPCR mediated mechanism but also dopaminergic D1, D2, D4 and D5 receptors [83], adenosine A1 and A2 receptors [84] and metabotropic glutamate receptors [85], among others, were characterized in this tissue.

In the study, G protein-coupled receptor kinases 2, 3 and 5 were expressed in different regions and cell populations of the chick retina. While immunoreactivity of GRK2 was found over all types of neurons of the retina and over both plexiform layers, immunolabeling for GRK3 was restricted to the inner portion of the retina, over the inner plexiform layer and amacrine and ganglion cell bodies. However, immunoreactivity for GRK5 was only found in amacrine and Muller glial cells bodies and processes [39].

6. Muscarinic receptors in avian trachea

Another study characterized a muscarinic receptor in chicken trachea controlling secretion of chlorides. In the study the chicken trachea was stimulated to secrete chloride ions by the application of acetyl choline and this was completely inhibited by bumetanide suggesting the presence of a functional muscarinic receptor in the avian trachea. In the study they classified the receptor subtype as M4, which probably is involved in ion transport on exocrine glands and mucosal cells [31].

7. Muscarinic receptors in avian gastrointestinal system

Characterization of muscarinic receptors in avian smooth muscles has been done by many researchers, especially in the ileum of chicken using functional and binding studies. Decades back, a contractile response to carbachol antagonized by atropine had been studied in the chick ileum [86]. In the functional studies, the affinities obtained exhibited good agreement with the existence of a functional M3 muscarinic receptor subtype in the ileum of chicken, however the findings were in direct contrast to the binding experiments, in which the single binding site appeared to be the muscarinic M2 receptor subtype. Hence, even though the contractile response was mostly due to a functional M3 receptor subtype, analysis of the competition binding curves suggested the presence of a uniform population of the muscarinic M2 receptor subtype also even though it did not contribute to the contractile response [28].

8. Muscarinic receptors in avian cardiovascular system

As mentioned above, initially the only available data on chicken muscarinic receptors was that of the M2 muscarinic receptor subtype. But many ex-vivo experiments have given proof for the existence of avian correlates in atria of chick for muscarinic M2 receptor [77], M3 receptors in atrium and ventricles [23] and M5 receptor subtype in embryonic chick heart and brain [24]. The potent muscarinic cholinergic antagonist 3 -quinuclidinyl benzylate (QNB) has been used to detect and quantify muscarinic receptors as early as day 3 *in ovo* in the developing chick heart [87]. The study found an exponential increase in 3 -quinuclidinyl benzylate (QNB) binding sites, which reduced at day 18 *in ovo.* However, the receptor density and subtype were not investigated in the above study.

Another study determined the effect of exposure of cardiomyocytes from chicken embryos for 3 days to the beta adrenoceptor agonist, isoproterenol. In the study, the 3 days exposure induced an increase in the level of muscarinic acetylcholine receptors by about 30% in chicken cardiomyocytes [88].

Another study found out the inotropic response of muscarinic acetyl choline receptors to the stimulation of isolated chick ventricular myocardium at various developmental stages. The study also pharmacologically characterized the receptor subtype involved in embryonic chick ventricles. Carbachol produced positive inotropy in embryonic chick ventricles at micromolar concentrations, whereas in hatched 1–3-day old chick ventricles it produced negative inotropy at nanomolar concentrations. However, in the 19–21-day-old embryos, neither positive nor negative inotropy was observed. Conclusions were made by comparing the pA_2 values that positive inotropy is most likely due to muscarinic M1 receptors and the negative inotropy is most likely mediated by muscarinic M4 receptors [22].

9. Muscarinic acetylcholine receptors in the avian salt gland

Unlike other vertebrate exocrine glands, the avian salt gland secretes an effluent that contains only trace amounts of protein or other macromolecular species, which makes it a unique model for the study of exocrine secretion of electrolytes [89]. This hypertonic secretion principally contains sodium and chloride ions in the rage of 500 to 900 mEq/l concentrations [15]. Administration of acetylcholine or methacholine in herring gulls stimulated salt gland secretion, while secretion in response to either a parenteral salt load or to a direct stimulation of the secretory nerve is blocked by injection of atropine, which suggests the role of muscarinic receptors responsible for its secretory function. In order to demonstrate and characterize these receptors in avian salt gland, radiolabeled muscarinic antagonist [H]quinuclidinyl benzilate ([^{3}H] QNB) was used in ducklings under fresh water and salt water conditions.

Characterization of these receptors using the radiolabeled antagonist, [^{3}H]QNB, showed them to be similar to muscarinic receptors from various mammalian sources, including rabbit iris, rabbit heart, rat parotid gland, and rat brain [90]. Regardless of conditions, since the DNA content of individual cells in the salt gland remains the same in case of salt stress, relating [^{3}H]QNB binding to DNA allows calculation of average number of receptors per cell. Upon conducting this calculation, it became evident that individual salt gland cells in salt water contains approximately three times as many muscarinic receptors as that of fresh water glands [15]. These results thus provide direct evidence for *de novo* synthesis of muscarinic cholinergic receptors during the plasma membrane hypertrophy that typifies the response of salt gland epithelial cells to chronic salt stress.

10. Muscarinic receptors in quail

The first report of muscarinic acetylcholine receptors in Japanese quail intestine was evaluated by recording the contractile responses of quail ileum to the agonist and agonist in presence of antagonists, also relaxant effect of muscarinic receptor antagonists with submaximal contraction of Ach using an isometric transducer. In the study, EC50 values of ACh increased in the presence of atropine (nonselective muscarinic antagonist) and pirenzepine (M1/M2 muscarinic antagonist) compared to EC50 value of ACh alone. Also, the EC50 value of Ach was higher in the presence of atropine when compared to EC50 of ACh in presence of solifenacin (M3 muscarinic antagonist). It was also found that EC50 of ACh was increased 3.48 times in presence of atropine, 2.65 times in presence of pirenzepine and 1.56 times in presence of solifenacin. These findings indicate that the muscarinic receptor subtypes responsible for contraction of small intestine in Japanese quail is contributed by both M2 and M3 muscarinic receptor subtypes, and it was substantiated using molecular studies which revealed the absence of M_1 receptor gene in Japanese quail and this finding is in accordance with the reports in chicken. The results of the study indicated that muscarinic receptors are distributed with the same propensity in quails like that of other avian and other mammalian species [34].

11. Conclusions

Several research have revealed that different bird species like chicken, pigeon and herring gulls have numerous functioning muscarinic receptors. The receptors in these species are mostly found in the central nervous system (dorsal root ganglia, basilar artery) and heart, as well as in sensory structures like the vestibular periphery and in avian salt glands respectively. Several studies have found them in the trachea, proventriculus and in smooth muscles of the intestinal tissue (ileum, rectum). The paper also reviews the existence of muscarinic receptors in quail ileum, a first report of its own in quail. Major receptor subtypes identified in avians are M2, M3, M4 and M5 except for M1 receptors present in dorsal root ganglion, atria and ventricles of heart and vestibular periphery. Even though, the muscarinic receptor subtypes in avians have been identified and characterized, the transduction mechanisms and functional contribution of each receptor subtypes has not been studied properly, which is a major shortcoming of researches in avian muscarinic receptors. For the goal of organizing the prospective neurophysiological and pharmacological research of cholinergic transmission in this species, it is crucial to establish the functional role of cholinergic systems in avians. However, in spite of the findings discussed here, rigorous studies are required in this field to further investigate the function and expression of mAChRs in avians.

Conflict of interest

The authors declare no conflict of interest.

Author details

Presannan Usha Aswathy[1], Suresh Narayanan Nair[1*], Basavapura Mahadevappa Sanjay[2] and Sanis Juliet[3]

1 Department of Veterinary Pharmacology and Toxicology, College of Veterinary and Animal Sciences, Thrissur, India

2 Safety Assessment, Syngene International Ltd, Bengaluru, India

3 Department of Veterinary Pharmacology and Toxicology, College of Veterinary and Animal Sciences, Wayanad, India

*Address all correspondence to: suresh@kvasu.ac.in; snn11@rediffmail.com

References

[1] Moroz LL, Romanova DY, Kohn AB. Neural versus alternative integrative systems: Molecular insights into origins of neurotransmitters. Philosophical transactions of the Royal Society of London. Series B, Biological sciences. 1821;**376**:2021. DOI: 10.1098/rstb.2019.0762

[2] Scarr E. Muscarinic receptors: Their roles in disorders of the central nervous system and potential as therapeutic targets. CNS Neuroscience & Therapeutics. 2012;**18**(5):369-379. DOI: 10.1111/j.1755-5949.2011.00249.x

[3] Peralta EG, Ashkenazi A, Winslow JW, Smith DH, Ramachandran J, Capon DJ. Distinct primary structures, ligand-binding properties and tissue-specific expression of four human muscarinic acetylcholine receptors. The EMBO Journal. 1987;**6**(13):3923-3929. DOI: 10.1002/j.1460-2075.1987.tb02733.x

[4] Jakubik J, El-Fakahany EE. Current advances in allosteric modulation of muscarinic receptors. Biomolecules. 2020;**10**(2):1-16. DOI: 10.3390/biom10020325

[5] Eglen RM. Overview of muscarinic receptor subtypes. Handbook of Experimental Pharmacology. 2012;**208**:3-28. DOI: 10.1007/978-3-642-23274-9_1

[6] Grassiolli S, Gravena C, de Freitas Mathias PC. Muscarinic M2 receptor is active on pancreatic islets from hypothalamic obese rat. European Journal of Pharmacology. 2007;**556**(1-3):223-228. DOI: 10.1016/j.ejphar.2006.11.022

[7] Wess J et al. M1-M5 muscarinic receptor knockout mice as novel tools to study the physiological roles of the muscarinic cholinergic system. Receptors and Channels. 2003;**9**(4):279-290. DOI: 10.1080/10606820308262

[8] Wess J, Liu J, Blin N, Yun J, Lerche C, Kostenis E. Structural basis of receptor/G protein coupling selectivity studied with muscarinic receptors as model systems. Life Sciences. 1997;**60**(13-14):1007-1014. DOI: 10.1016/S0024-3205(97)00041-6

[9] Matsui M et al. Multiple functional defects in peripheral autonomic organs in mice lacking muscarinic acetylcholine receptor gene for the M3 subtype. Proceedings of the National Academy of Sciences of the United States of America. 2000;**97**(17):9579-9584. DOI: 10.1073/pnas.97.17.9579

[10] Van Koppen CJ, Kaiser B. Regulation of muscarinic acetylcholine receptor signaling. Pharmacology & Therapeutics. 2003;**98**(2):197-220. DOI: 10.1016/S0163-7258(03)00032-9

[11] Bradley P, Horn G. Imprinting: A study of cholinergic receptor sites in parts of the chick brain. Experimental Brain Research. 1981;**41**:121-123

[12] Wachtler K. And acetylcholinesterase in vertebrate brains of different

[13] Dietl MM, Cortés R, Palacios JM. Neurotransmitter receptors in the avian brain. II. Muscarinic cholinergic receptors. Brain Research. 1988;**439**(1-2):360-365. DOI: 10.1016/0006-8993(88)91495-3

[14] Tietje KM, Goldman PS, Nathanson NM. Cloning and functional analysis of a gene encoding a novel muscarinic acetylcholine receptor expressed in chick heart and brain.

The Journal of Biological Chemistry. 1990;**265**(5):2828-2834. DOI: 10.1016/s0021-9258(19)39876-x

[15] Hootman SR, Ernst SA. Characterization of muscarinic acetylcholine receptors in the avian salt gland. The Journal of Cell Biology. 1981;**91**(3 I):781-789. DOI: 10.1083/jcb.91.3.781

[16] Guo JZ, Chiappinelli VA. Muscarinic receptors mediate enhancement of spontaneous GABA release in the chick brain. Neuroscience. 1999;**95**(1):273-282. DOI: 10.1016/S0306-4522(99)00391-7

[17] Tata AM, Tripiciano A, Filippini A, Biagioni S, Augusti-Tocco G. Muscarinic receptors modulate intracellular calcium level in chick sensory neurons. Brain Research. 2000;**866**(1-2):65-72. DOI: 10.1016/S0006-8993(00)02225-3

[18] Matsumoto F, Watanabe Y, Obi T. Physiology, Endocrinology, and Reproduction Characterization of 5-hydroxytryptamine-induced contraction and acetylcholine-induced relaxation in isolated chicken basilar artery Responsiveness to 5-HT, and Effect of Methiothepin or Ketanserin on 5-HT-ind. 2011:1158-1165

[19] Jeck D, Lindmar R, Loffelholz K, Wanke M. Subtypes of muscarinic receptor on cholinergic nerves and atrial cells of chicken and guinea-pig hearts. 1998;**93**:357-366

[20] Zendehdel M, Lankarani Mohajer L, Hassanpour S. Central muscarinic receptor subtypes (M1 and M3) involved in carbacol-induced hypophagia in neonatal broiler chicken. The International Journal of Neuroscience. 2020;**130**(2):204-211. DOI: 10.1080/00207454.2019.1667792

[21] Brehm G, Lindmar R, Lffeiholz K. Archives of Pharmacology Inhibitory and excitatory muscarinic receptors modulating the release of acetylcholine from the postganglionic parasympathetic neuron of the chicken heart*. 1992;**346**:375-382

[22] Nouchi H, Kaeriyama S, Muramatsu A, Sato M, Hirose K, Shimizu N. Full paper muscarinic receptor subtypes mediating positive and negative inotropy in the developing chick ventricle. Journal of Pharmacological Sciences. 2007;**82**:75-82

[23] Gadbut AP, Galper JB. A novel M3 muscarinic acetylcholine receptor is expressed in chick atrium and ventricle. The Journal of Biological Chemistry. 1994;**269**(41):25823-25829. DOI: 10.1016/s0021-9258(18)47321-8

[24] Creason S, Tietje KM, Nathanson NM. Isolation and functional characterization of the chick M5 muscarinic acetylcholine receptor gene. Journal of Neurochemistry. 2000;**74**(2):882-885. DOI: 10.1046/j.1471-4159.2000.740882.x

[25] Yin GC, Gentle A, McBrien NA. Muscarinic antagonist control of myopia: A molecular search for the M1 receptor in chick. Molecular Vision. 2004;**10**:787-793

[26] Mcbrien NA, Arumugam B, Gentle A, Chow A, Sahebjada S. The M4 muscarinic antagonist MT-3 inhibits myopia in chick: Evidence for site of action. Ophthalmic & Physiological Optics. 2011;**31**(5):529-539. DOI: 10.1111/j.1475-1313.2011.00841.x

[27] Kitazawa T, Taneike T, Ohga A. Functional characterization of neural and smooth muscle motilin receptors in the chicken proventriculus and ileum. Regulatory Peptides. 1997;**71**(2):87-95. DOI: 10.1016/S0167-0115(97)01024-0

[28] Darroch S, Irving HR, Mitchelson FJ. Characterisation of muscarinic receptor subtypes in avian smooth muscle. European Journal of Pharmacology. 2000;**402**(1-2):161-169

[29] Fischer AJ, Kinnon LAMC, Nathanson NM, Stell WK. Identification and localization of muscarinic acetylcholine receptors in the ocular tissues of the Chick. 1998;**284**:273-284

[30] Zagvazdin Y, Fitzgerald MEC, Reiner A. Role of muscarinic cholinergic transmission in Edinger-Westphal nucleus-induced choroidal vasodilation in pigeon. Experimental Eye Research. 2000;**70**(3):315-327. DOI 10.1006/exer.1999.0791

[31] Winding B, Bindslev N. Characterization of a muscarinic receptor controlling Cl- secretion in hen trachea. American Journal of Physiology-Cell Physiology. 1990;**258**(6):27-26. DOI: 10.1152/ajpcell.1990.258.6.c982

[32] Li GQ, Correia MJ. The inhibitory effect of carbachol on pigeon inwardly rectifying potassium channel pKir expressed in transfected tsA-201 cells and native type II vestibular hair cells. Neuroscience Abstracts (On-Line). 2005:47.7

[33] Shiina T, Takewaki T. Purinergic control of the quail rectum : Modulation of adenosine 5 0-triphosphate-mediated contraction with acetylcholine. 2007;**82**:246-251. DOI: 10.1016/j.rvsc.2006.07.006

[34] Sanjay BM, Nair SN, Juliet S, Megha M, Shijin MS, Suraj SV, et al. First report of functional identification of muscarinic receptors in the small intestine of Japanese quail (Coturnix coturnix japonica). Journal of Experimental Biology and Agricultural Sciences. 2020;**8**(1):71-75. DOI: 10.18006/2020.8(1).71.75

[35] De Azevedo LC, Zizemer JR, Häckl LPN, Marino-Neto J, Paschoalini MA. Muscarinic cholinergic receptor blockade impairs free fatty acid mobilization during fasting in pigeons (*Columba livia*). Journal of Comparative Physiology. B, Biochemical, Systemic, and Environmental Physiology. 2002;**172**(2):115-123. DOI: 10.1007/s00360-001-0233-0

[36] Kohler EC, Messer WS Jr, Bingman VP. Evidence for muscarinic acetyicholine receptor subtypes in the pigeon telencephalon. The Journal of Comparative Neurology. 1995;**362**(2):271-282

[37] Khan KM, Drescher MJ, Hatfield JS, Khan A-M, Drescher DG. Muscarinic receptor subtypes are differentially distributed in the rat cochlea. Neuroscience. 2002;**111**(2):291-302

[38] Li GQ, Kevetter GA, Leonard RB, Prusak DJ, Wood TG, Correia MJ. Muscarinic acetylcholine receptor subtype expression in avian vestibular hair cells, nerve terminals and ganglion cells. Neuroscience. 2007;**146**(1):384-402. DOI: 10.1016/j.neuroscience.2007.02.019

[39] De Almeida Gomes CP, Ventura ALM. Localization of G protein-coupled receptor kinases (GRKs) in the avian retina. Brain Research Bulletin. 2004;**63**(6):499-507. DOI: 10.1016/j.brainresbull.2004.04.010

[40] de Azua IR, Gautam D, Guettier J-M, Wess J. Novel insights into the function of β-cell M3 muscarinic acetylcholine receptors: Therapeutic implications. Trends in Endocrinology and Metabolism. 2011;**22**(2):74-80

[41] Olianas MC, Dedoni S, Onali P. Involvement of store-operated Ca2+ entry in activation of AMP-activated protein kinase and stimulation of glucose uptake by M3 muscarinic acetylcholine receptors in human neuroblastoma cells. Biochimica et Biophysica Acta (BBA) - Molecular Cell Research. 2014;**1843**(12):3004-3017

[42] Shabani S, Foster R, Gubner N, Phillips TJ, Mark GP. Muscarinic type 2 receptors in the lateral dorsal tegmental area modulate cocaine and food seeking behavior in rats. Neuroscience. 2010;**170**(2):559-569

[43] Veenman CL, Reiner A. The distribution of GABA-containing perikarya, fibers, and terminals in the forebrain and midbrain of pigeons, with particular reference to the basal ganglia and its projection targets. The Journal of Comparative Neurology. 1994;**339**(2):209-250

[44] Weiner DM, Levey AI, Brann MR. Expression of muscarinic acetylcholine and dopamine receptor mRNAs in rat basal ganglia. Proceedings of the National Academy of Sciences. 1990;**87**(18):7050-7054

[45] Ehlert FJ. Pharmacological analysis of the contractile role of M 2 and M 3 muscarinic receptors in smooth muscle. Receptors and Channels. 2003;**9**(4):261-277

[46] Harris DA, Falls DL, Johnson FA, Fischbach GD. A prion-like protein from chicken brain copurifies with an acetylcholine receptor-inducing activity. Proceedings of the National Academy of Sciences of the United States of America. 1991;**88**(17):7664-7668. DOI: 10.1073/pnas.88.17.7664

[47] Reiner A et al. Revised nomenclature for avian telencephalon and some related brainstem nuclei. The Journal of Comparative Neurology. 2004;**473**(3):377-414

[48] Jarvis ED et al. Avian brains and a new understanding of vertebrate brain evolution. Nature Reviews. Neuroscience. 2005;**6**(2):151-159

[49] Karakuyu D, Herold C, Güntürkün O, Diekamp B. Differential increase of extracellular dopamine and serotonin in the 'prefrontal cortex'and striatum of pigeons during working memory. The European Journal of Neuroscience. 2007;**26**(8):2293-2302

[50] Lissek S, Güntürkün O. Out of context: NMDA receptor antagonism in the avian'prefrontal cortex'impairs context processing in a conditional discrimination task. Behavioral Neuroscience. 2005;**119**(3):797

[51] Sarter M, Bruno JP. Cortical cholinergic inputs mediating arousal, attentional processing and dreaming: Differential afferent regulation of the basal forebrain by telencephalic and brainstem afferents. Neuroscience. 1999;**95**(4):933-952

[52] Sarter M, Parikh V, Howe WM. nAChR agonist-induced cognition enhancement: Integration of cognitive and neuronal mechanisms. Biochemical Pharmacology. 2009;**78**(7):658-667

[53] Bozkurt A et al. Distributions of transmitter receptors in the macaque cingulate cortex. NeuroImage. 2005;**25**(1):219-229

[54] Herold C et al. The receptor architecture of the pigeons' nidopallium caudolaterale: An avian analogue to the mammalian prefrontal cortex. Brain Structure & Function. 2011;**216**(3):239-254. DOI: 10.1007/s00429-011-0301-5

[55] Krames ES. The role of the dorsal root ganglion in the development of neuropathic pain. Pain Medicine (United States). 2014;**15**(10):1669-1685. DOI: 10.1111/pme.12413

[56] Scott SA. Sensory Neurons: Diversity, Development, and Plasticity. USA: Oxford University Press; 1992

[57] Tata AM, Plateroti M, Cibati M, Biagioni S. C holinergic markers are expressed in developing and mature neurons of Chick dorsal root ganglia. 1994;**255**:247-255

[58] Tata AM, De Stefano ME, Bernardini N, Placidi F, Biagioni S, Augusti-Tocco G. Characterization and immunocytochemical localization of muscarinic acetylcholine receptors in chick dorsal root ganglia. Life Sciences. 1997;**13**(60):1198

[59] Boyd RT, Jacob MH, McEachern AE, Caron S, Berg DK. Nicotinic acetylcholine receptor mRNA in dorsal root ganglion neurons. Journal of Neurobiology. 1991;**22**(1):1-14

[60] Vilaro MT, Wiederhold K-H, Palacios JM, Mengod G. Muscarinic cholinergic receptors in the rat caudate-putamen and olfactory tubercle belong predominantly to the m4 class: in situ hybridization and receptor autoradiography evidence. Neuroscience. 1991;**40**(1):159-167

[61] Bernardini N, De Stefano ME, Tata AM, Biagioni S, Augusti-Tocco G. Neuronal and non-neuronal cell populations of the avian dorsal root ganglia express muscarinic acetylcholine receptors. International Journal of Developmental Neuroscience. 1998;**16**(5):365-377. DOI: 10.1016/S0736-5748(98)00038-0

[62] Pannese E. Fine Structure of Neurons, Nerve Processes and Neuroglial Cells. New York Thieme: Neurocytol; 1994

[63] Mirsky R, Jessen KR. The neurobiology of Schwann cells. Brain Pathology. 1999;**9**(2):293-311

[64] Cuthbertson S, White J, Fitzgerald MEC, Shih Y-F, Reiner A. Distribution within the choroid of cholinergic nerve fibers from the ciliary ganglion in pigeons. Vision Research. 1996;**36**(6):775-786

[65] Fitzgerald ME, Vana BA, Reiner A. Control of choroidal blood flow by the nucleus of Edinger-Westphal in pigeons: A laser Doppler study. Investigative Ophthalmology & Visual Science. 1990;**31**(12):2483-2492

[66] Zagvazdin YS, Fitzgerald ME, Sancesario G, Reiner A. Neural nitric oxide mediates Edinger-Westphal nucleus evoked increase in choroidal blood flow in the pigeon. Investigative Ophthalmology & Visual Science. 1996;**37**(4):666-672

[67] Bungardt E et al. Characterization of muscarinic receptors mediating vasodilation in Guinea-pig ileum submucosal arterioles by the use of computer-assisted videomicroscopy. European Journal of Pharmacology. 1992;**213**(1):53-61

[68] Loke KE, Sobey CG, Dusting GJ, Woodman OL. Cholinergic neurogenic vasodilatation is mediated by nitric oxide in the dog hindlimb. Cardiovascular Research. 1994;**28**(4):542-547

[69] Wessler I, Kirkpatrick CJ, Racké K. Non-neuronal acetylcholine, a locally acting molecule, widely distributed in biological systems: Expression and function in humans. Pharmacology & Therapeutics. 1998;**77**(1):59-79

[70] Nomura J, Hosoi T, Okuma Y, Nomura Y. The presence and functions of muscarinic receptors in human T cells: The involvement in IL-2 and IL-2 receptor system. Life Sciences. 2003;**72**(18-19):2121-2126

[71] Kawashima K, Fujii T. Expression of non-neuronal acetylcholine in lymphocytes and its contribution to the regulation of immune function. Frontiers in Bioscience. 2004;**9**(3):2063-2085

[72] Eglen RM. Muscarinic receptor subtypes in neuronal and non-neuronal cholinergic function. Autonomic & Autacoid Pharmacology. 2006;**26**(3):219-233

[73] McBrien NA, Moghaddam HO, Reeder AP. Atropine reduces experimental myopia and eye enlargement via a nonaccommodative mechanism. Investigative Ophthalmology & Visual Science. 1993;**34**(1):205-215

[74] Luft WA, Ming Y, Stell WK. Variable effects of previously untested muscarinic receptor antagonists on experimental myopia. Investigative Ophthalmology & Visual Science. 2003;**44**(3):1330-1338

[75] Stone RA, Lin T, Laties AM. Muscarinic antagonist effects on experimental chick myopia. Experimental Eye Research. 1991;**52**(6):755-758

[76] Cottriall CL, Truong H-T, McBrien NA. Inhibition of myopia development in chicks using himbacine: A role for M4 receptors? Neuroreport. 2001;**12**(11):2453-2456

[77] Tietje KM, Nathanson NM. Embryonic chick heart expresses multiple muscarinic acetylcholine receptor subtypes. Isolation and characterization of a gene encoding a novel m2 muscarinic acetylcholine receptor with high affinity for pirenzepine. The Journal of Biological Chemistry. 1991;**266**(26):17382-17387

[78] Premont RT, Inglese J, Lefkowitz RJ. Protein kinases that phosphorylate activated G protein-coupled receptors. The FASEB Journal. 1995;**9**(2):175-182

[79] Sterne-Marr R, Benovic JL. Regulation of G protein-coupled receptors by receptor kinases and arrestins. Vitamins and Hormones. 1995;**51**:193-234

[80] Inglese J, Freedman NJ, Koch WJ, Lefkowitz RJ. Structure and mechanism of the G protein-coupled receptor kinases. The Journal of Biological Chemistry. 1993;**268**(32):23735-23738

[81] Zhao X, Huang J, Khani SC, Palczewski K. Molecular forms of human rhodopsin kinase (GRK1). The Journal of Biological Chemistry. 1998;**273**(9):5124-5131

[82] Zhao X, Yokoyama K, Whitten ME, Huang J, Gelb MH, Palczewski K. A novel form of rhodopsin kinase from chicken retina and pineal gland 1. FEBS Letters. 1999;**454**(1-2):115-121

[83] Nguyen-Legros J, Versaux-Botteri C, Vernier P. Dopamine receptor localization in the mammalian retina. Molecular Neurobiology. 1999;**19**:181-204

[84] de Carvalho RP, De Mello FG. Adenosine-elicited accumulation of adenosine 3′, 5′-cyclic monophosphate in the chick embryo retina. Journal of Neurochemistry. 1982;**38**(2):493-500

[85] Thoreson WB, Witkovsky P. Glutamate receptors and circuits in the vertebrate retina. Progress in Retinal and Eye Research. 1999;**18**(6):765-810

[86] Choo LK, Mitchelson F, Napier P. Differences in antagonist affinities at muscarinic receptors in chick and Guinea-pig. Journal of Autonomic Pharmacology. 1988;**8**(3):259-266

[87] Sastre A, Gray DB, Lane MA. Muscarinic cholinergic binding sites in the developing avian heart. Developmental Biology. 1977;**55**(1):201-205. DOI: 10.1016/0012-1606(77)90332-3

[88] Reithmann C, Panzner B, Werdan K. Distinct pathways for β-adrenoceptor-induced up-regulation of muscarinic acetylcholine receptors and inhibitory G-protein α-subunits in chicken cardiomyocytes. Naunyn-Schmiedeberg's Archives of Pharmacology. 1992;**345**(5):530-540. DOI: 10.1007/BF00168944

[89] Fänge R, Schmidt-Nielsen K, Robinson M. Control of secretion from the avian salt gland. The American Journal of Physiology Content. 1958;**195**(2):321-326

[90] Yamamura HI, Snyder SH. Muscarinic cholinergic binding in rat brain. Proceedings of the National Academy of Sciences. 1974;**71**(5):1725-1729

Chapter 3

Central Nicotinic and Muscarinic Receptors in Health and Disease

Yousef Tizabi, Bruk Getachew, Vassiliy Tsytsarev, Antonei B. Csoka, Robert L. Copeland and Thomas Heinbockel

Abstract

Without acetylcholine (ACh) no skeletal muscle contraction, no preganglionic sympathetic or parasympathetic activity can be obtained. This can result in dysregulation of cardiac, respiratory, gastrointestinal, and renal functions as well as disruption of fluid secretion from various glands such as tears, saliva, digestive juices, sweat, and milk. Importantly, ACh deficiency in the brain can have severe cognitive consequences. The action of ACh is mediated by two distinct classes of receptors, namely the muscarinic (mAChRs), which are G-protein coupled (metabotropic) receptors and nicotinic receptors (nAChRs), which are ligand-gated ion channels (ionotropic receptors). The focus of this chapter is on interaction of these two distinct receptor classes and its implication in health and disease. Thus, following a brief description of ACh actions and its central circuitry, an update on mAChRs and nAChRs and how their interaction may impact neuropsychiatric/neurodegenerative diseases will be provided. Moreover, potential novel therapeutic intervention based on these interactions, particularly in relationship to Alzheimer's and Parkinson's diseases will be touched upon.

Keywords: acetylcholine, nicotinic receptors, muscarinic receptors, glial cells, neuroinflammation

1. Introduction

It is now 100 years since acetylcholine (ACh), described as "vagus stuff" by Otto Loewi has been recognized as the first discovered neurotransmitter. This discovery was based on an ingenious experiment where the exposure of a second heart to the media obtained from the electrical stimulation of the vagus nerve of the first heart, resulted in slowing of the second heart, similar to the effect observed by vagal stimulation of the first heart. ACh is now recognized as a critical neurotransmitter at various vital sites such as neuromuscular junction, autonomic ganglia and the brain or the central nervous system (CNS).

Without ACh no skeletal muscle contraction, no preganglionic sympathetic or parasympathetic activity can be obtained. This can result in dysregulation of cardiac, respiratory, gastrointestinal, and renal functions as well as disruption of secretion from various glands such as tears, salvia, digestive juices, sweat and milk. Moreover, since ACh is also the neurotransmitter at the adrenal medulla, its absence at this site would prevent the release of adrenaline, an essential hormone in regulating the fight-fright response. Importantly, lack of ACh in the brain can have severe cognitive consequences.

Acetylcholine, as the name implies, is made up from two substances, an acetyl group (derived from glucose) and choline, a nutrient derived from foods such as egg yolks, soy and legumes. Choline is also synthesized by the liver. ACh synthesis is catalyzed by choline acetyltransferase (ChAT), the presence of which in a neuron implies that ACh is used as a neurotransmitter by that neuron. A distinguished feature of ACh in comparison with other neurotransmitters is that its action in the synapse is readily terminated by the enzyme acetylcholinesterase (AChE), in contrast to the reuptake mechanism prevalent with other neurotransmitters. Upon the action of AChE, ACh is broken down into acetate and choline, where the latter is taken up for re-use by the nerve. Inhibition of AChE by insecticides or nerve gases can result in accumulation of ACh. Excess ACh at the neuromuscular junction would cause depolarization of the post-synaptic cell and paralysis. Death from the nerve gas is primarily due to excess secretion and respiratory paralysis. On the other hand, some AChE inhibitors (AChEIs) can be used as therapeutic agents in diseases where ACh transmission is inadequate. This includes myasthenia gravis where AChEIs raise the level of ACh in the neuromuscular junction, and improve muscle activation, contraction, and strength, or in neurological disease such as Alzheimer's disease (AD).

The action of ACh is mediated by two distinct classes of receptors, namely the muscarinic (mAChRs) and nicotinic receptors (nAChRs). The focus of this chapter is on interaction of these 2 distinct receptor classes and its implication in health and disease. Thus, following a brief description of ACh actions and its central circuitry, an update on mAChRs and nAChRs and how their interaction may impact neuro-psychiatric/neurodegenerative diseases will be provided. Moreover, potential novel therapeutic intervention based on these interactions will be touched upon.

2. Brain ACh pathways and their significance

An extensive local interneuron network in brain areas involved in motor, cognitive and reward activities such as the striatum, nucleus accumbens, and neocortex utilize ACh as a neurotransmitter. In addition, cholinergic pathways connecting the basal forebrain, a complex of 4 cholinergic nuclei that project to: cerebral cortex, hippocampus, amygdala and the olfactory bulb, are critical in regulating cognition, motivation, hedonic state and reinforcement. Cholinergic input to the substantia nigra pars compacta (SNpc), ventral tegmental area (VTA), thalamus and hypothalamus, areas critical in regulating motor, reward and endocrine systems are provided by the pedunculopontine nucleus (PPN) and laterodorsal tegmental nucleus (LDTN) [1]. Moreover, lateral habenula (LatH), part of a complex nucleus which connects the midbrain to the limbic forebrain and uses ACh, has received considerable attention because of its potential role in cognition and in the pathogenesis of various psychiatric disorders. The medial habenula (MedH), which can be further subdivided into a dorsal region containing non-cholinergic excitatory neurons such as tachykinin and substance P and a ventral region containing dense cholinergic neurons, has recently been investigated more thoroughly. It is now believed that cholinergic projections of MedH is involved in mood regulation as well as drug addiction and that manipulation of this system may be therapeutically exploited [2].

Thus, extensive trajectories throughout the brain, such as cortical connections mediating decision making and planning; projections to the hippocampus and amygdala influencing attention, memory, fear, and stress responses; mesolimbic pathways affecting response to reward; hypothalamic system controlling homeostatic responses such as thermoregulation, food intake, and sleep, all utilize ACh as a neurotransmitter. Furthermore, cholinergic system plays an important role in facilitating synaptic plasticity and neuronal development [1]. For these reasons, the cholinergic systems, particularly, the basal forebrain complex, PPN and LDTN have been extensively studied in relation to age-related progressive neurodegenerative diseases such as Alzheimer's disease (AD) and PD [1].

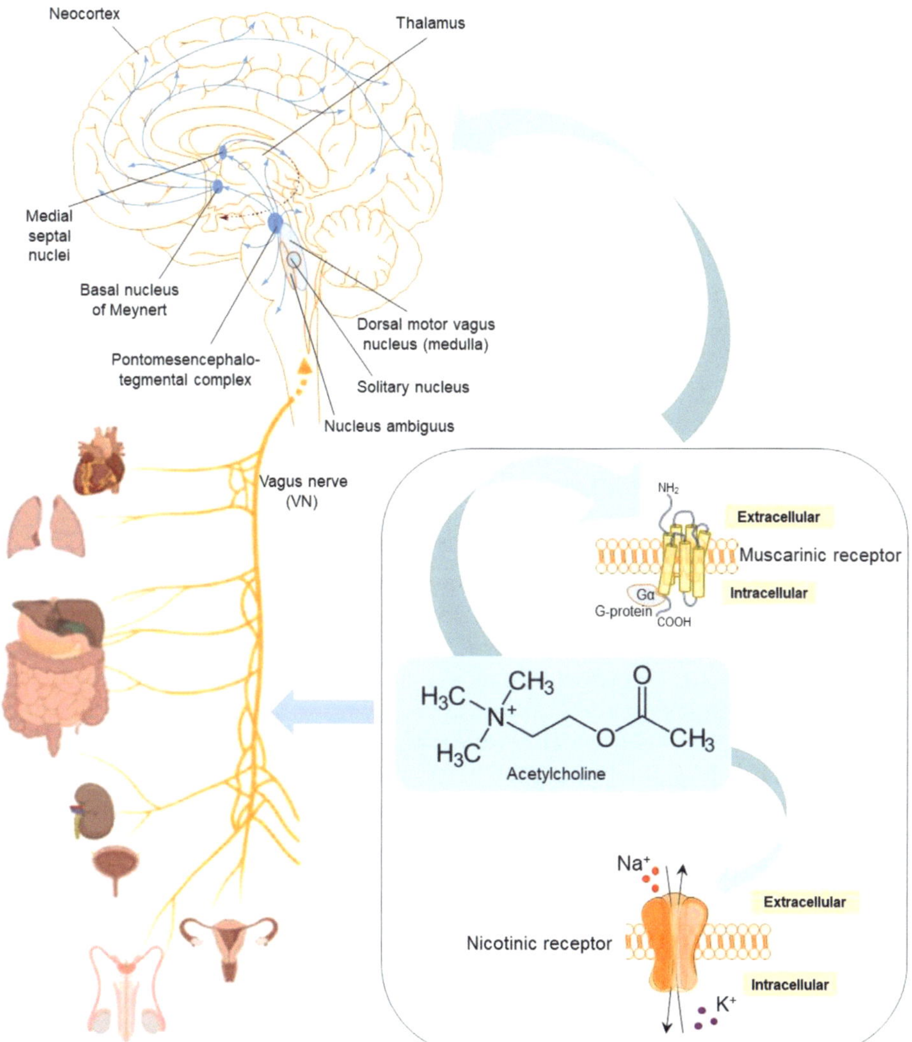

Figure 1.
Simplified schematic diagram depicting central cholinergic system as well as its interaction with the peripheral organs. The afferent and efferent connections of the vagus nerve with the heart, lung, gastrointestinal (GI) tract, kidney and the gonadal system are highlighted. Moreover, the mediators of acetylcholine (ACh) actions (i.e., muscarinic and nicotinic receptors) and their structural composition (i.e., G-protein coupled receptor vs. ligand-gated ion channels) are distinctly shown in the insert.

It is also of relevance to note that the cholinergic projections, in general, have a modulatory, rather than strictly excitatory or inhibitory effects on other neuronal systems. As mentioned earlier, ACh action is mediated by both nicotinic and muscarinic receptors, which interact at both pre- and post-synaptic junctions. A major emphasis of this chapter is to provide an up-to-date understanding of this complex interaction (**Figure 1**).

3. ACh receptors

As mentioned above, the cholinergic system is involved in a wide variety of functions in peripheral as well as in CNS. ACh is the neurotransmitter widely distributed in CNS, used by motor neurons at the neuromuscular junction, and by sympathetic and parasympathetic preganglionic neurons in the autonomic nervous system (ANS), by the parasympathetic innervated organs and select sympathetic-innerved organs including sweat glands, the piloerector muscle (responsible for skin hair to stand up), and other smooth muscles such as irises, which control the diameter of the pupils. In all these, ACh effect is mediated by activating two distinct types of receptors: muscarinic acetylcholine receptors (mAChRs) and nicotinic acetylcholine receptors (nAChR) that differ in both structure and function but share common neuronal circuits. Moreover, these two receptors may co-localized in the same or in different cells, where they can interact with each other. For example, nAChRs in ganglionic cells may modulate the functions of mAChRs in target organs such as smooth muscle, cardiomyocytes, epithelium, and exocrine cells. Below, following brief descriptions of the two classes of receptors, their role in relation to the neurodegenerative diseases will be the focus.

3.1 Muscarinic acetylcholine receptors (mAChRs)

There are five subtypes of mAChRs: M1, M2, M3, M4 and M5 which are G-protein coupled receptors (GPCRs) responsive to the agonist muscarine with equal affinity [3]. Depending on the subtype of mAChR stimulated, distinct signaling pathways are activated. For example, stimulation of the M2 and M4 subtypes, leads to activation of inhibitory G-protein (Gi) which results in inhibition of cyclic AMP (cAMP) and consequent effects downstream. In contrast, activation of M1, M3 and M5 subtypes is generally coupled to a (Gq) which activates phospholipase C that leads to the formation of inositol 1,4,5-trisphosphate (IP3) and diacylglycerol (DAG). IP3 causes mobilization of Ca^{2+} from intracellular stores, while DAG activates protein kinase C (PKC) isozymes [4], which can phosphorylate a multitude of downstream molecules that exert tissue-specific functions [5]. In addition, activation of mAChRs can modulate several types of ion channels and currents. For example, Ca^{2+} currents can be suppressed by M1 and M2 receptors in the mouse and M1 and M4 receptors in the rat, whereas M1 receptors can suppress M-type K^+ current in the rat [6]. Furthermore, MAP kinases and small GTPases, such as Rho and Rac proteins, are also activated by mAChRs [4]. It is worth mentioning that Gq and Gs are designation for stimulatory, whereas Gi signifies inhibitory effect on second messenger such as cAMP.

3.2 Brain distribution of mAChRs

The predominant mAChR subtypes expressed in the cortex of adult brain are: M1(40%), M2 (37%) and M4 (15%). In the hippocampus, however, 36%, 33% and

27% represent M1, M2 and M4, respectively. As mentioned earlier, M1 receptors are found throughout the brain with highest concentrations in cortical regions and the hippocampus. Cortical M1 receptors, most dominant in cortical layers III and V/VI in pyramidal neurons are primarily located post-synaptically and are associated with excitatory synapses. M2 receptors, on the other hand, are highly localized in the nucleus basalis and occipital cortex, and with lesser density in the hippocampus, caudate putamen, and other cortical regions. M2 receptors are located both pre- and post-synaptically in the cortex, where the latter is present in a subset of glutamatergic synapses and GABAergic interneurons. The presynaptic M2 receptors are located on the axons of symmetric synapses and function as autoreceptors. An autoreceptor is a type of receptor located in the nerve membrane and serves as part of a negative feedback loop in signal transduction and is only sensitive to the neurotransmitters released by the neuron on which it is located. M3 receptors have similar distribution to that of M1 but with a much lower level of expression. Like M1, M3 receptors also are present in cortical pyramidal neurons and glial cells. In contrast, M4 receptors are highest in the caudate putamen and are often associated with dopaminergic neurotransmission. M5 receptors are present in very low levels in the hippocampus, substantia nigra, and ventral tegmental area.

3.3 Function of mAChRs

mAChRs shape neuronal and local network processing abilities, and depending on the network involved, affect cognitive functions including learning and memory. For example, AD related-cognitive impairment is associated with reduced muscarinic cholinergic activity, although ascribing specific contribution of individual mAChR subtypes to a specific cognitive performance is not tenable due to heterogeneous distribution of mAChR subtypes within the brain [7]. Knockout studies show that mAChRs functions are subtype dependent. For instance, in paradigms requiring hippocampal processing, M1−/− animals appear to have normal learning and memory [8, 9], suggesting other AChRs may be at play. However, in paradigms thought to require interactions between the hippocampus and cortex, M1−/− animals show deficits [10]. These deficits are thought to be analogous to working memory impairment which may require communication between the two regions and possibly through recruitment of M1 receptors. Thus, mAChRs, with their potential to modulate cognition, have stimulated a high degree of interest as a therapeutic target.

3.4 Nicotinic acetylcholine receptors (nAChRs)

Advances in this area have identified various subtypes of nAChRs with distinct anatomical, physiological, and pharmacological characteristics. These ionotropic classified receptors act by directly regulating the opening of a cation channel in the neuronal membrane. It is important to note that nAChRs present at the neuromuscular junction differ from those in autonomic ganglia which are also different from those occurring in CNS, as each has its distinct subunit structure. Neuronal nicotinic receptors are primarily alph4-beta2 or homomeric alpha7 subtypes. Extensive research on these receptors has led to the suggestion of therapeutic potential for selective nicotinic receptor agonists in various neuropsychiatric and neurodegenerative disorders, including PD, AD, schizophrenia, depression, pain as well as smoking cessation [11–13].

3.5 Brain distribution of nAChRs

The nAChRs are distributed in various brain regions including the ventral tegmental area, hippocampus, prefrontal cortex, amygdala, and nucleus accumbens. The two most abundant nAChRs, α7 nAChRs (α-bungarotoxin sensitive) and α4β2 (α-bungarotoxin insensitive), are localized in the brainstem, cerebellum, mesencephalic structures, limbic system and cortex. The α4β2, the first to be pharmacologically characterized, constitutes the principal nAChR subtype in the cortex, striatum, superior colliculus, lateral geniculate nucleus and cerebellum. The second abundant nAChR subtype, α7 subunit-containing receptors, have high expression in the cortex, hippocampus and subcortical limbic regions, and are expressed at low levels in the thalamic regions and basal ganglia. Although α7 nAChRs anatomical distribution differ markedly from α4β2, the two co-localize in some areas such as in the superficial layer of the superior colliculus. nAChRs are located in pre- and postsynaptic regions well as in extra-synaptic locations. Specially, receptors containing the β2 subunit are located diffusely throughout the membrane of the neuron.

3.6 Function of nAChRs

Studies from receptor subunit knockout mice have shown that brain nAChRs are not essential for survival or for the execution of basic behaviors. They are, however, critical for control of several complex behaviors and maintenance of mental health. Modulation of presynaptic nAChRs and, less frequently, postsynaptic nAChRs is responsible for large number of behaviors and brain functions including locomotion, nociception, anxiety, learning and memory, as well as behaviors associated with drug abuse and mental illness. Moreover, stimulation of presynaptic nAChRs receptors promotes neurotransmitter release including dopamine (DA), norepinephrine (NE), serotonin (5HT), glutamate, GABA and ACh.

4. AChRs and inflammation

4.1 Role of nicotinic receptors

It is now recognized that there exists a cholinergic anti-inflammatory pathway that acts primarily but not exclusively, through nicotinic acetylcholine receptors. In particular, such pathway has been well characterized in peripheral organs such as spleen where splenic nerve stimulation leads to release of norepinephrine, which in turn, causes release of ACh, where an anti-inflammatory effect is produced [14]. This is because abundant nicotinic (α7 nAChR) are expressed in variety of immune cells including B cells, T cells and macrophages. Activation of these receptors can suppress production of pro-inflammatory cytokines such as TNF- α, IL-1, IL-6 without affecting the anti-inflammatory cytokines such as IL-10. Indeed, several animal models such as sepsis, ischemia–reperfusion, and pancreatitis, which are associated with elevated levels of pro-inflammatory cytokines, show improvement by vagal stimulation. It is believed that this improvement is mediated via activation of α7 nAChRs on macrophages [14, 15]. This contention is further supported by the finding that α7 nAChRs deficient mice show increased endotoxin-induced TNF-α production, which do not respond to electrical vagal stimulation. Because nicotine is a potent activator of nAChRs, including α7 subtype, it was proposed as a potential intervention in control of cytokine storm associated with COVID-19 [11].

4.2 Role of muscarinic receptors

A role for mAChRs in inflammatory response is also evident. However, it appears that the direction of effect, at least in some tissues such as airway smooth muscle, is opposite to that of nicotinic receptor stimulation, in that mAChRs stimulation, leads to pro-inflammatory, rather than anti-inflammatory consequence [16]. But, in intestinal epithelial cells mAChRs play an important role in the maintenance of homeostasis. Notedly, these cells in addition to absorbing essential nutrients, also prevent the entry of foreign antigens (micro-organisms and undigested food) through mucus secretion and epithelial barrier formation. Since disruption of the intestinal epithelial homeostasis exacerbates inflammation, mAChR agonists may be of therapeutic potential in diseases associated with such disruptions such as inflammatory bowel disease [17]. However, it is important to note that unselective activation of mAChRs may have deleterious effects on intestinal epithelial barrier function. This is because subtypes of mAChRs may have distinct and in some cases opposing effects [17]. Additionally, a comprehensive understanding of the ACh network throughout the intestinal tissue, including the relationship between muscarinic and nicotinic receptors, is yet to be elucidated. In the following section, we concentrate of central interactions between these 2 distinct classes of receptors.

5. Nicotinic-muscarinic receptor interactions

5.1 Central Co-localization of nicotinic and muscarinic receptors

The overlapping distributions of nAChRs and mAChRs in the brain is well characterized. Up to 90% of central cholinergic neurons express both types of receptors as seen in several thalamic nuclei, the interpeduncular nucleus, the superior colliculus, and the cerebral cortex. These overlaps signify important interactions. For example, in striatal DA system, nAChRs and mAChRs counteract each other's effects, in that DA efflux is stimulated by nAChRs activation or in contrast, by inhibition of mAChRs [18]. Similarly, in corpus striatum, ACh released from cholinergic interneurons can activate α4β2 nAChRs mediating release of GABA. This evoked release, on the other hand, can be negatively modulated by M4 mAChRs co-expressed on the same GABAergic terminals [19]. Therefore, it appears that some of the counteractive effects of nAChRs and mAChRs observed in peripheral organs (described above, see 4.2) also extend to the brain. However, exploitation of such interactions is yet to be fully explored.

5.2 Desensitization of nAChRs and effect on mAChRs

Chronic nicotine exposure is associated with a long-lasting desensitization of nAChRs, which is both time- and concentration-dependent. In desensitization state, an intrinsic property of brain nAChRs, the receptor does not respond to nicotine or ACh. Although desensitization may lead to upregulation of nAChRs (an increase in the number of receptors), the overall response is diminished. This desensitization of nAChRs results in hypersensitization of mAChRs, stimulation of which by a muscarinic agonist can lead to electroencephalogram seizures, behavioral convulsions, tremors and inhibition of spontaneous locomotor activity [20]. Moreover, hypersensitivity of mAChRs does not occur after nAChR recovery from desensitization. In addition to affecting mAChRs, desensitization of nAChRs also affects the activities of other systems. For example, desensitized nAChRs reduce GABA release from interneurons leading to disinhibition of pyramidal cells in hippocampus and cerebral cortex [21]. Conversely, activation of interneuron nAChRs enhances GABA release which inhibits pyramidal cells in these areas.

Interestingly, chronic administration of a mAChR antagonist such as scopolamine results in upregulation of cortical nAChRs [22]. Thus, it appears that inhibition of one receptor class such as nAChRs via desensitization, or inhibition of the other receptor class such as mAChRs via administration of an antagonist, results in upregulation or hypersensitization of the second receptor class, possibly as a compensatory mechanism. This fits with the findings that show administration of nAChRs and mAChRs antagonists together significantly decreases the development of kindled seizures in the amygdala, whereas either drug alone is ineffective [23].

6. Excess ACh

Overall, excess ACh in synaptic cleft results in overstimulation of nicotinic or muscarinic receptors, which in turn, result in activation of the glutamatergic system and the development of seizures [24]. Other central effects include cognitive impairments (discussed below), as well as motivational, arousal and attentional problems. Indeed, this is the mechanism of toxicity induced by organophosphorus compounds, including nerve gases, whereby inhibition of AChE causes accumulation of ACh in the synapse. Aside from central site, peripheral accumulation of ACh may lead to dysregulation in heart contraction, blood pressure, decrease heart rate, increase glandular secretion including saliva, tear, sweat and digestive juices, increase in urination frequency, visual disturbance and importantly, inhibition of muscle contraction due to nicotinic receptor desensitization. Generation of reactive oxygen species (ROS), neuroinflammation are other causes of neuropathies.

Atropine, a mAChR antagonist, is the primary antidote used to counter organophosphate poisoning. However, specific cases of inhibition of nAChRs by atropine have also been reported [25]. In order to overcome the effect of organophosphates on nicotinic receptors, which can result in muscle weakness, fasciculation and paralysis, pralidoxime (2-PAM) also should be given, as 2-PAM tends to reactivate AChE. Interestingly, 2-PAM may also have some muscarinic inhibition, although such effect is not clinically significant and hence necessity of co-administration with atropine [25].

In addition, patients with seizures are given benzodiazepine (BZ), which stimulate GABAAR. Since BZs are of limited efficacy in overall organophosphate toxicity, it is suggested that antagonizing the hyperactivity of the glutamatergic system could provide an even more efficacious approach in protecting the brain from permanent damage. This may be further helped by adding an anticholinergic agent [24].

7. Nicotinic-muscarinic interaction in memory and cognition

Cholinergic system is implicated in memory and cognition functions. ACh is diffusely released throughout the cortex during periods of high attentional demand which could act on nAChRs and mAChRs, both of which are critically important in cognitive processes such as learning, memory, attention, and other higher brain functions. Manipulation of these receptors exert distinguishable effects on different cognitive functions. For instance, working memory is required for remembering information that varies unpredictably in time and/or in content. It refers to the cognitive system that holds information temporarily and is important for reasoning and decision-making. In contrast, reference memory is a long-term memory that deals with the recall of the content and place of an event.

Both mAChRs and nAChRs modulate not only working and reference memory, but other indices of cognitive functions such as attention and learning. For example, muscarinic M1 receptors in prefrontal cortex [26, 27], and nicotinic receptors, particularly α7 and α4β2 receptors, modulate firing of dorsolateral prefrontal cortex excitatory networks that underlie working memory function [28, 29]. Moreover, muscarinic M1 receptors, may also interact with glutamatergic NMDA receptors in regulation of working memory [30].

Several pharmacological studies have attempted to disentangle the role of nAChRs and mAChRs in different cognitive domains. Blocking mAChRs by scopolamine causes impairment of different aspects of memory processing such as acquisition of new information, consolidation of memory, sustained attention, reaction time, as well as visual discrimination [31, 32]. Antagonism of nAChRs, on the other hand, affects declarative memory (immediate and delayed word recall and delayed recognition), attention and psychomotor function (reaction time), suggesting that attention and psychomotor (reaction time) may be mediated by both mAChRs and nAChRs. This contention is further supported by the findings that blockade of both mAChRs and nAChRs impair working memory (spatial and non-spatial), short-term memory, declarative memory, sustained visual attention, and psychomotor function far more than each antagonist alone [33]. Similar observations were also seen in object and spatial n-back working memory performance where simultaneous antagonism of mAChRs and nAChRs produced greater effect than each antagonist alone [34].

In another cognitive domain, inspection time (IT), a measure of early visual information processing speed, it was determined that the efficiency of visuospatial attention is sensitive to manipulation by both nAChRs and mAChRs. Simultaneous antagonism of both mAChRs and nAChRs induced larger impairments in early information processing (in an inspection time task) than antagonism of either receptor alone [31]. Curiously, impairments in early information processing, a hallmark feature of diverse neuropsychiatric disorders including schizophrenia and AD, may contribute to impairments in other cognitive domains including attention and memory. It is of relevance to note that age-related alterations in mAChR and nAChR interactions also occur [35]. Hence, several lines of evidence implicate a dysfunction of the cholinergic system in cognitive dysfunctions including in AD. This topic is further discussed below, mainly in relationship to AD and PD.

8. Glial cells

There are greater number of glial cells than neurons (between five and ten times more) in CNS. Different types of cells comprise glia. For example, astrocytes, radial glia, and oligodendroglia are of neural origin, whereas microglia are differentiated blood monocytes during ontogeny, where neurons develop first, and glial cells develop later. Glial cells exert a profound effect on neuronal development by providing trophic support essential for neuronal survival and are involved in neuronal

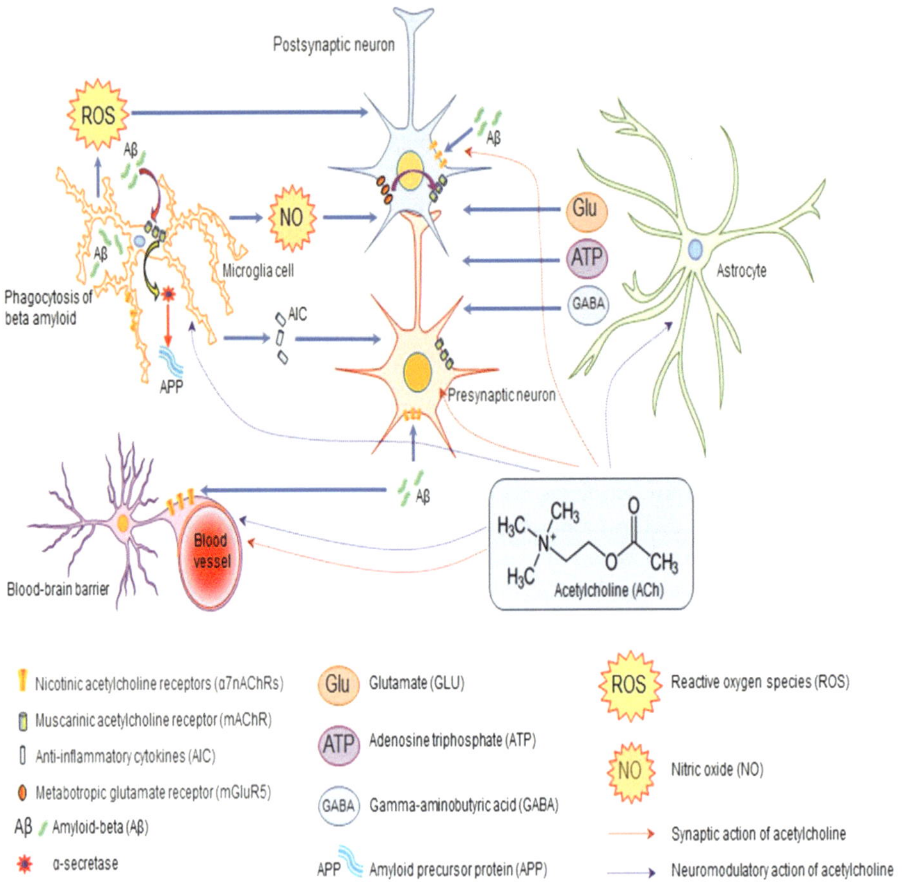

Figure 2.
Schematic diagram depicting the influence of ACh as well as the roles of mAChRs and nAChRs (primarily alpha7 subtype) in microglia and astroglia modulation of pre- and post-synaptic neurons. Note the production of ROS and NO by microglia as well as interaction of Aβ with both nicotinic and muscarinic receptors.

migration, axon, and dendrite outgrowth, and in synaptogenesis (**Figure 2**) [36]. Below, the role of microglia and astrocytes in AD pathology and the influence of cholinergic system on them is discussed in more detail.

8.1 Alzheimer's disease (AD): microglia

AD, the most common age-related neurodegenerative disease, is characterized by cognitive decline in people over 65 years old. Pathologically, AD is presented with amyloid-β protein (Aβ) deposition (plaques), abnormal phosphorylation aggregation of the microtubule-associated protein tau (tangles), neuroinflammation, oxidative stress, and synaptic dysfunction. Neuroinflammation is underscored by microglial reaction and increased cytokine production. Microglia are also major sources of free radicals such as superoxide and nitric oxide in the brain. Microglia are considered the innate immune cells of the CNS and act as brain macrophages. They are mainly found in the subventricular and subgranular zone, where under physiological conditions self-renew over an organism's entire lifespan. Microglia are not uniformly distributed throughout the brain. A large number is present in the hippocampal dentate gyrus, substantia nigra, and parts of the basal ganglia. Interestingly, olfactory telencephalon in mice has the largest microglial population.

Microglia differ in size and ramification patterns within and between different histological layers of the cerebellar cortex. Substantia nigra contains the largest proportion of microglia (about 12%) compared to 5% in the cortex and corpus callosum. This regional heterogeneity is attributed to the residential environment, especially interactions with neurons or neural progenitor cells, as well as intrinsic mechanisms. Microglia are critical for regulation of the neuronal network as they support the development, maintenance, homeostasis, and repair of the brain by wiping out cell debris and phagocytizing viruses and bacteria. There are several stages in microglia morphology and function. For example, during the resting state, microglia are sensitive to environmental stimuli such as stress that can activate aberrant microglia functioning and lead to neurodegenerative and psychiatric disorders. Thus, it is critical to recognize microglial heterogeneity in identifying microglia-selectively therapies and uncover the underlying mechanisms that activate the reparative and regenerative functions of microglia [37, 38].

Pro-inflammatory microglia (M1-activated state) secrete proinflammatory cytokines such as tumor necrosis factor-α (TNF-α), interleukin (IL)-1β, IL-6, and inducible nitric oxide synthase (iNOS), which typically lead to dysfunction following chronic activation. In contrast, neuroprotective microglia (M2 state) phagocytose cell debris and misfolded proteins, promote tissue repair and reconstruction of the extracellular matrix and support neuron survival mediated by neurotrophic factors [39].

AD is also associated with changes in neurovascular unit NVU, a structural and functional complex that maintains microenvironmental homeostasis and metabolic balance in CNS. Microglia are one of the most important components of the NVU. In AD, microglia may also cause blood–brain barrier (BBB) breakdown due to loss of pericytes. Pericytes are cells present at intervals along the walls of capillaries and are important for blood vessel formation, maintenance of BBB, regulation of immune cell entry into CNS and control of brain blood flow. Thus, BBB breakdown can lead to infiltration of peripheral white blood cells into CNS, abnormal contraction of cerebral vessels and neurovascular uncoupling (**Figure 2**) [40].

Family history is the second strongest risk factor following advanced age. Twin and family studies indicate that genetic factors are estimated to play a role in at least 80% of AD [41]. Moreover, autosomal dominant and late onset sporadic AD share a common pathophysiology [42]. Numerous sporadic AD risk genes including apolipoprotein E (ApoE) and complement receptor 1 (CR1), are highly expressed in microglia and affect microglial phagocytosis of amyloid-beta peptides. Actually, during the early stages of AD, microglia may provide protection against amyloid accumulation but in advanced AD stage they promote neuropathology. Indeed, approximately two-thirds of AD patients risk single nucleotide polymorphisms that are exclusively or dominantly expressed in microglia. Furthermore, AD is associated with increased microglial proliferation. It is noteworthy that microglia exert a “double-edged sword” effect involving neuroprotective or neurotoxic functions dependent on contextual factors as well as disease stage. Thus, at the early stage of AD, microglia are involved in clearance of Aβ and tau proteins from the brain, whereas in the later stages of AD, sustained microglial activation leads to chronic pro-inflammatory state, associated with increase production of pro-inflammatory cytokines, reactive oxygen species (ROS), and dysfunctional lysosomal deposits, all of which adversely affect neuronal survival by promoting protein aggregation and hence causing neuronal damage. Altogether, the findings suggest that further characterization of microglia and its detailed role in neurodegeneration, can lead to novel therapeutic targets for AD [38, 39, 43].

8.2 AD: astrocytes

It is believed that astrocytes are involved in many vital cognitive functions, including learning and memory. Moreover, astrocytes through production of antioxidant and anti-inflammatory proteins are involved in CNS protection. They also clean the extracellular environment and facilitate neuronal communication and help in maintenance of homeostasis. However, full exploitation of glial system as potential development of novel drugs and techniques to reverse oxidative stress and/or excess of inflammation that occurs in many CNS diseases, remains to be investigated (**Figure 2**) [44].

In contrast to microglia, astrocytes are brain cells that mainly control metabolic and redox homeostasis. Due to their swift response to brain pathology in the initial stages of the disease, their activation and differentiation are implicated in the pathogenesis of multiple neurodegenerative diseases, including AD [45]. Astrocytes play an important role in synaptic function, K+ buffering, BBB maintenance and neuronal metabolism. For example, BBB disruption occurs in the early stages of AD, which is associated with cognitive decline and might accelerate the disease progression. Reactive astrocytes denote astrocytes undergoing morphological, molecular and functional remodeling in response to pathological stimuli. During AD progression, reactive astrogliosis occur. For this reason, it has been suggested that manipulation of astrocytes and/or astrocytic biomarkers could be developed in diagnosis and/or treatment of AD (**Figure 2**) [46, 47].

Blood biomarkers have been investigated for the diagnosis, prognosis, and monitoring of AD. Although Aβ and tau are primarily blood biomarkers, recent studies have identified other reliable candidates such as glial fibrillary acidic protein (GFAP), an astrocytic cytoskeletal protein that can be detected in blood samples. Indeed, it has been suggested that GFAP levels can be used to detect early-stage AD. This is based on observations where GFAP level in the blood was higher in the Aβ-positive group than in the negative groups, and in individuals with AD or mild cognitive impairment (MCI) compared to the healthy controls [47]. Thus, astrocyte activation, accompanied by high levels of GFAP is often observed in AD patients. This elevated GFAP occurs around Aβ plaque, indicative of elevated phagocytosis. Structural alterations in AD astrocytes including swollen endfeet and soma shrinkage contribute to disruption in vascular integrity at capillary and arterioles levels. Astrocyte endfeet enwrap the entire vascular tree within CNS where they perform important functions in regulating BBB, cerebral blood flow, nutrient uptake, and waste clearance [48]. Like microglia in AD, astrocytes also are skewed into proinflammatory and oxidative profiles with increased secretions of vasoactive mediators inducing endothelial junction disruption and immune cell infiltration [49]. Regarding biomarkers, astrocytic α7nAChR levels or activity, was recently proposed as a marker since this receptor subtype is implicated in instigation and potentiation of early Aβ pathology. The same receptors could provide a target for therapeutic intervention in AD [46].

Recently, it has been proposed that the term “type III diabetes (T3DM)” be used in conjunction with AD as both conditions share similar molecular and cellular features. For example, T3DM is associated with insulin resistance and cognitive decline (memory deficits) in elderly individuals. Since astrocytes are involved in brain metabolism (e.g., glucose metabolism, lipid metabolism), neurovascular coupling, synapses, and synaptic plasticity, targeting them might be promising in alleviating neurodegeneration in these patients [50].

8.3 ACh-AChRs: microglia

As mentioned above, neuroinflammation linked to glial function has been demonstrated to participate in the pathogenesis of AD (**Figure 2**). Moreover, anti-inflammatory and neuroprotective properties of ACh in several neurodegenerative disorders was also alluded to. More recently, specific influence of ACh on neuroinflammation and neurodegeneration in AD was investigated. It was reported that microglia played a key role in lipopolysaccharide (LPS)-induced hippocampal neuronal toxicity and that ACh, via activation of α7nAChR provided anti-inflammatory and neuroprotective effects. Furthermore, in neuron–microglia co-cultures, LPS increased the expression of pro-inflammatory factors, including iNOS, interleukin-1α, and tumor necrosis factor-α, and decreased expression of neurotrophic factors such as insulin-like growth factor-1, and neuronal apoptosis. However, ACh, via the action of α7nAChR on microglia, inhibited LPS-induced inflammatory response and provided neuroprotection, which was further enhanced by promoting microglial neurotrophic factor production [51]. Targeting microglia in age-related cognitive decline and AD, and bearing in mind the heterogeneity of microglia in these conditions and how pharmacological agents could target specific microglial states, has been recently reviewed [52]. Infiltration of immune cells into the brain might play a role in detrimental effects of activated microglia as this can lead to T-cell infiltration, which can induce tauopathy, another marker of AD neuropathology. Interestingly, drugs or antibodies that can result in death of microglia, have shown protection against brain atrophy in mice [53].

Microglia may contain both nAChRs and mAChRs. It is believed that a subpopulation of microglia that express functional mAChRs play a role in stroke and AD. These microglia tend to expand in these conditions, which are sensitive to blockers of protein synthesis and correlate with an upregulation of the M3 receptor subtype. Thus, carbachol, a mAChR agonist acts as a chemoattractant for microglia and reduces their phagocytic activity [54]. In addition to M3 receptor upregulation, there is an increased expression of major histocompatibility complex (MHC)-I and MHC-II. MHC molecules plays an important role in alerting the immune system to virally infected cells [55].

As mentioned above, nAChRs presence in microglia and consisting primarily of α7nAChR provide anti-inflammatory and neuroprotective effects. Hence, manipulation of microglial nAChRs and mAChRs may offer a new therapeutic strategy in neurodegenerative diseases in general, and AD, in particular.

8.4 ACh-AChRs: astrocytes

ACh and AChRs are present in the brain before synaptogenesis occurs and are believed to be involved in neuronal maturation. Astrocytes express mAChRs whose activation stimulates a robust intracellular signaling that regulate neurite outgrowth in hippocampal neurons, a system intimately involved in cognitive function. In fact, stimulation of astrocytes induces the release of permissive factors that accelerate neuronal development [36]. Moreover, it was recently demonstrated that M1 muscarinic receptors in astrocytes mediate cholinergic regulation of adult hippocampal neurogenesis [56].

In CNS, as mentioned earlier, ACh is mainly present in interneurons. However, at least two important cholinergic pathways have also been identified. One is the cholinergic projection from the nucleus basalis of Meynert (in the basal forebrain) to the forebrain neocortex and associated limbic structures, degeneration of which is one of the pathologies associated with AD. The other is a projection from the medial septal and diagonal band region to limbic structures, commonly referred to as the septo-hippocampal pathway that is also involved in memory formation [57]. In both cases, both nAChRs and mAChRs mediate the effects of ACh, where nicotinic agonists including nicotine, have been shown to improve working memory, whereas muscarinic agonists may be more relevant to improvement of reference memory [58, 59].

AD patients have a substantial reduction in nAChRs in the cortex and hippocampus. Recently, using local cholinergic lesions it was possible to manipulate the cholinergic system more finely to determine the role of AChRs as well as nicotinic-muscarinic receptor interactions that can either synergize or antagonize the behavioral outcomes. Therefore, potential utility of combining selective nAChR subtypes as well selective mAChRs on memory and cognition warrants further investigation [60, 61]. It is noteworthy that along such selective agonists, manipulation of vesicular ACh transporter should also be considered [62].

That astrocytes express nAChRs was mentioned above. These receptors, predominantly α7nAChR and regulating calcium signaling, are likely mediators of nicotine's effects on morphological and functional changes of the astrocytes [63]. Interestingly, nicotine does not induce reactive astrocytosis even at high concentrations (10 μM) as determined by cytokine release and GFAP expression in-vitro. In vivo also, nicotine induces a change in the volume of astrocytes in the prefrontal cortex, CA1 of the hippocampus, and the substantia nigra. These and other findings indicate potential use of nicotine in neurodegenerative diseases including AD [10, 64, 65]. However, mode of nicotine administration appears to be an important factor in its therapeutic application. It is argued that pulsatile (e.g., via inhalation or nasal spray), rather than continuous administration of nicotine (e.g., via patch) would likely be effective for providing neuroprotection in any neurodegenerative disease [66].

Muscarinic M1 and M4 ACh receptors are also highly pursued drug targets for neurological diseases including AD. However, due to high sequence homology in M1-M5 mAChRs, selective targeting of any subtype through endogenous ligand binding site has been difficult to achieve. Recent discovery of highly subtype selective mAChR positive allosteric modulators has provided a new frontier in novel drug development. However, due to side effects, where M1 mAChR over-activation can have detrimental consequences, a drug candidate may need to exhibit a biased signaling profile. In this regard, recent studies in mice suggest that allosteric modulators for the M1 mAChR that bias signaling toward specific pathways may be therapeutically important [67].

9. Parkinson's disease (PD)

PD, the second most common progressive neurodegenerative disorder, is associated with loss of dopaminergic neurons in SNpc that leads to striatal DA deficiency. This loss of dopaminergic neurons results in motor deficits characterized by akinesia, rigidity, resting tremor, and postural instability as well as non-motor symptoms that might also involve other neurotransmitter systems. The non-motor symptoms may involve emotional changes such as apathy, anxiety and depression, mild or severe cognitive impairment, sleep disturbance (either insomnia or hypersomnia), autonomic dysfunction affecting bladder (frequent and urgent need to urinate), blood pressure (orthostatic hypotension), sweat glands (excessive sweating), sensory dysfunction (feeling of pain, loss of acuity in vision and olfaction), gastrointestinal disturbance (constipation and/or nausea) as well as "social symptoms" such as inability to recognize other's verbal and nonverbal cues or produce facial expression.

The neuronal degeneration in PD likely involves several cellular and molecular events including accumulation of misfolded proteins aggregates, failure of protein clearance pathways, mitochondrial damage, oxidative stress, neuroinflammation, immune dysregulation, apoptosis, excitotoxicity, Ca++ dysregulation, autophagy and dysbiosis. Implicated in neuronal degeneration are also mutations in genes such as Parkin RBR E3 ubiquitin protein ligase (PARK2), Leucine-rich repeat kinase 2 (LRRK2), PTEN-induced putative kinase 1(PINK1), Parkinson disease protein 7 (PARK7), and Synuclein Alpha (SNCA) as well as polymorphism in DRD2 gene Taq1A (DRD2Taq1A) and DA receptor D2 (DRD2).

PD is believed to be a multifactorial disease, where both genes and environmental factors play a crucial role. Old age, starting at 60 years is considered the primary risk factor for PD. This risk increases with advanced age. In addition, it is postulated that exposure to environmental toxicants such as pesticides, herbicides, and heavy metals may increase the risk of PD.

Serendipitously, it was discovered in the early 1980's that administration of 1-methyl-4-phenyl-1,2,3,6-tetrahydropyridine (MPTP), an underground laboratory preparation, could result in motor symptom typical of PD. This discovery was the impetus to use MPTP, a potent analog of meperidine, an opioid analgesic, as a pharmacological model of PD. MPTP is metabolized into the neurotoxin MPP^+ (1-methyl-4-phenylpyridinium), which is not only substrate for DA transporter (DAT) but is also a potent mitochondrial complex-I inhibitor. Because MPP^{++} selectively damages dopaminergic cells in SNpc, it is commonly used to investigate the mechanism of neurotoxicity and/or development of novel therapeutics. Similarly, rotenone, a pesticide that selectively inhibits mitochondrial complex I, is used to generate animal models of PD. Finally, exposure to heavy metals such as manganese or iron have also been implicated in PD etiology. Interestingly, reduction of iron content was associated with a remarkable improvement of the motor and non-motor deficits in an MPTP-induced monkey model of PD [12, 13].

Oxidative stress has also been linked with the onset and/or progression of several neurodegenerative diseases including PD. In fact, overproduction of reactive oxygen species correlates with AD, Huntington's disease, amyotrophic lateral sclerosis, multiple sclerosis (MS) and PD [68]. It is noteworthy that oxidative stress and neuroinflammation are linked and affect one another [69].

9.1 Treatment modalities for PD

Despite tremendous effort in understanding the causes and/or treatment of PD, no cure is yet available. Current medications are geared toward replenishing central DA transmission, which can only offer symptomatic relief without dealing with the neurodegenerative aspect of the disease. In this case, DA replacement or use of DA agonists to directly stimulate DA receptors are the mainstay of therapy. Unfortunately, these therapies lose efficacy after few years and in some cases such as with L-Dopa treatment, the side effects, commonly referred to L-Dopa-induce dyskinesia can be just as bad if not worse than PD symptoms. Thus, to prolong the efficacy of L-Dopa, it is combined with carbidopa. Alternatively, DA agonists such as pramipexole or ropinirole are used first. Other options include use of monoamine oxidase inhibitors, such as selegiline or rasagiline, or catechol-O-methyltransferase (COMT) inhibitors, such as entacapone and tolcapone. Combination therapy using multiple drugs with various mechanism of action may also be applied. Non-pharmacological interventions may include physical and occupational therapy, repetitive transcranial magnetic stimulation (rTMS), and in specific circumstances neurosurgery (i.e., deep brain stimulation), which is reserved for those who meet well-defined criteria. Moreover, significant effort is devoted in developing regenerative treatments in the form of autologous or stem cell-derived grafts as well as viral gene therapies designed to replace the function of the neurons that have been lost. Thus, as our knowledge of contributing factors and their mechanisms become more clear, potential development of novel therapies also become a reality [12, 13].

9.2 ACh: PD

The cholinergic neurons of the mesopontine tegmental area and the basal forebrain send projections throughout the brain, regulating many discrete functions. Along with dopaminergic loss, cholinergic dysfunction also plays a substantial role in many PD symptoms such as cognitive impairment, gait problems, freezing of gait, falls, REM sleep behavior disorder (RBD), depression, visual hallucination, psychosis, and olfactory impairment. Thus, cholinergic dysfunction in PD could be contributing to a specific phenotype. This contention is further supported by the finding that a combination of RBD and a history of falls was able to predict combined thalamic and cortical cholinergic deficits. Nonetheless, further elucidation of cholinergic dysfunction, particularly in early stages of the disease is warranted [1]. Below, an update of our current knowledge regarding cholinergic receptors and PD is provided.

9.3 mAChRs: PD

It is now well-accepted that the striatum is the primary input structure of the basal ganglia, which participates in motivational and goal-directed behaviors. Basal ganglia output is controlled by local cholinergic interneurons (ChIs) and dopaminergic afferents. In general, the release of the neurotransmitters DA and ACh, acting through their respective receptors, elicits opposite effects on medial spiny neurons (MSNs). MSNs constitute 90–95% of all striatal neurons, while the remaining population consists of local ChIs and GABAergic interneurons in the striatum. Interestingly, a novel receptor-receptor interaction (i.e., heteromerization) between DA D2 receptor (D2R) and the muscarinic acetylcholine M1 receptor (M1R) was observed. This D2R-M1R complex coordinates a sophisticated interplay between the dopaminergic and cholinergic neurotransmission systems. Based on the existence of this heteromer within the striatum the use of anticholinergics drugs in the treatment of PD was suggested. Indeed, it was demonstrated that an M1R-selective antagonist could potentiate the antiparkinsonian-like efficacy of an ineffective D2R-selective agonist in a rodent model of experimental parkinsonism. Overall, the novel D2R-M1R heteromer could serve as a specific drug target to alleviate motor deficits in PD but with less side effects compared to other drugs [70].

Although giant, aspiny ChIs only represent 1–3% of striatal neurons, they are responsible for the highest concentration of ACh in the brain and interact with DA inputs to regulate motor function. ChIs possess an intrinsic firing activity referred to as autonomous pacemakers which modulate the activities of neuronal afferents. ChIs effects are mediated by both mAChRs and nAChRs. As mentioned earlier, the excitatory M1-like receptors (M1R, M3 R and M5R) transduce their signals through Gq/11proteins, whereas the inhibitory M2-like receptors (M2 R and M4R) are coupled to Gi/o proteins. The complexity of the striatal circuitry is underscored by the variety of DARs, mAChRs and nAChRs, their subcellular location in ChIs and MSNs as well as their interaction [70].

Due to the development of improved pharmacological agents targeting specific mAChR subtypes, the interest to modulate striatal function by anticholinergic drugs has been renewed in recent years. This is due to the findings that pharmacological blockade of mAChR subtypes, specifically M1R and M4R, can significantly add to other antiparkinsonian treatments. On the other hand, wild-type mice treated with M1R-selective agonist (i.e., telenzepine) had reduced anxiety-like behaviors. Moreover, mice deficient in M1R- exhibit an increased locomotor activity as well as elevated extracellular striatal DA levels. These mice, however, do not exhibit impairment in contextual fear condition, a test of hippocampal-dependent learning. Thus, M1R antagonist can be of benefit in motor impairments, whereas M1R agonist can have anxiolytic and, in some cases, (see above) cognitive enhancement effects. Moreover, M1R antagonists may suppress D2R-MSNs more efficiently than D1R-MSNs, through their interaction with potassium channels. Interestingly, striatal D2R-M1R formation might result in further differentiation of M1R signalization between the striato-pallidal and striato-nigral neurons. Additional support for reciprocal interaction between D2Rs and M1Rs is provided by the findings that systemic administration of scopolamine (i.e., non-selective mAChR antagonist) and benztropine (i.e., moderate M1R-selective antagonist) reduce the affinity of raclopride and spiperone (both D2R antagonists) for D2R in monkey brains [70].

Thus, it may be suggested that the dopaminergic-cholinergic imbalance, which is seen in most movement disorders, may be normalized by a combination of selective D2R agonist and M1R antagonist [70].

9.4 nAChRs: PD

The cholinergic system, particularly nAChRs are essential in modulating the striatal cells regulating cognitive and motor functions. Thus, nAChRs stimulation reduces neuroinflammation and facilitates neuronal survival, neurotransmitter release, and synaptic plasticity. PD is associated with loss of striatal nAChRs, which may aggravate the loss of dopaminergic neurons in this area, leading to pathological consequences. Additionally, nAChRs activation may also stimulate other brain cells supporting cognitive and motor functions [71].

Furthermore, the impairments in DA release observed in various animal models of PD (e.g., 6-OHDA lesioned rodents), appear to be exacerbated by loss of nAChRs activation. This suggests that DAergic imbalance may be ameliorated by nicotinic agonists and hence, nicotinic receptors may offer therapeutic targets for PD. In this regard, several in-vitro and in-vivo studies including primates and genetically modified mice have shown protective effects of nicotine against neuronal damage and/or neurotoxicity induced by 6-OHDA, MPTP, rotenone, methamphetamine, glutamate and β-amyloid. These effects are mediated via selective nAChR subtypes containing β2 and α7 subunits. Protective effects of nicotine against endogenous substances such as salsolinol and aminochrome that selectively damage dopaminergic cells have also been observed. More recently, protective effects of nicotine against toxicity induced by iron and manganese were also observed in cell culture. Interestingly, nicotinic cholinergic system may also play a role in L-Dopa-induced dyskinesias. Finally. an inverse relationship between PD incidence and any form of nicotine intake such as cigarette smoking, smokeless tobacco, exposure to environmental tobacco smoke or even from a dietary source such as peppers, also suggest a therapeutic potential for nicotine in PD. Hence, targeting nicotinic cholinergic receptors could be a novel intervention in PD. Nicotine's effects are likely to involve suppression of pro-inflammatory cytokines and stimulation of neurotrophic factors as well as suppression of oxidative stress [12, 13].

10. Importance of mode of nicotine administration

Several human studies have assessed the effects of nicotine gum or patch in PD, most of which have not yielded positive results. The negative finding in these trials is likely due to the mode of administration of nicotine. Thus, it is very important to consider the route of nicotine administration, where its subdermal administration via patch may not achieve the desirable nAChR stimulation that is obtained via pulsatile nicotine administration (e.g., via inhalation). The very complex dynamic interaction of nicotine with its receptors, where initial stimulation can be followed by rapid and differential desensitization of receptor subtypes, must be critically considered in experimental paradigms so that maximal therapeutic outcome may be obtained. It may be concluded therefore, that pulsatile stimulation of specific nAChRs in selective brain regions such as the nigrostriatal pathway is critical for the therapeutic efficacy of nicotine or nicotinic agonists in PD. Pulsatile stimulation of central nicotinic receptors may be achieved by currently available nicotine inhaler of nicotine nasal spray. The necessity of pulsatile stimulation may explain the negative outcome of nicotine patch in PD trials. A recent clinical study using oral administration of nicotine (pulsatile), reported positive effects of nicotine on falls and freezing gait in PD. Furthermore, pulsatile nicotine preparations in forms of inhalers or nasal spray are available and approved by FDA for smoking cessation and could be re-purposed for PD pending evaluation of their effectiveness in clinical trials. In addition, pulsatile nicotine administration may also be helpful in improving non-motor symptoms (e.g., depression or cognitive decline) that are commonly associated with PD [12, 13].

11. AD-PD-MS (multiple sclerosis)

In addition to the co-morbid manifestation of neuropsychiatric disorders with neurodegenerative diseases, potential co-morbid occurrence of neurodegenerative diseases such as AD and PD also exists [72]. This might not be very surprising given that the neurobiological substrates of one neurogenerative disease such as mitochondrial dysfunction, oxidative stress and inflammation may be very similar to another disease, except that the anomalies may be confined to specific brain areas and/or circuitries in different diseases. However, when there is an overlap or cross-over of circuitries, similar phenotypes could be manifested. For example, correlation between cholinergic system alterations, oxidative stress-and neuroinflammation in MS has been noted. MS is an autoimmune and demyelinating disease of the central nervous system, characterized by leucocytes infiltration, demyelination, axonal degeneration and neuronal death. As a result of disrupted central communication, different symptoms including vision loss, pain, fatigue, and impaired coordination may be manifested.

The role played by ACh in MS has been recently investigated. Cholinergic alterations may contribute to the dysregulated inflammatory processes of MS [73, 74]. Whether muscarinic or nicotinic receptor manipulation may be of therapeutic potential in MS also, needs to be further investigated.

12. Conclusion

In summary, ACh has maintained its importance in etiology and progression of various neurodegenerative diseases. Although the relevance of mAChRs and their exploitation was the predominant mode of cholinergic intervention in various disorders, including neurodegenerative diseases, the advent of nicotinic receptors and their prominent role in many important CNS functions, including cognitive behaviors such as learning, and memory has opened novel therapeutic potentials. This is not only applicable to neurodegenerative diseases such as AD and PD but also to neuropsychiatric disorders such as depression and schizophrenia. Moreover, significant interaction between these 2 distinct classes of receptors occurs. For example, as depicted in **Figure 2**, Aβ, a culprit protein in AD interacts with both receptors albeit at different locations and different cells (e.g., neuronal vs. glial). Despite notable advancements in our knowledge of these receptors, the complexity of cholinergic system in general, and nicotinic system in particular, requires further investigation on specific role of receptor subtypes in health and disease. Notedly, it is argued that pulsatile administration of nicotine or nicotinic agonists-modulators should be considered in any neurodegenerative and/or neuropsychiatric disease. This is due to the complex pharmacokinetic and pharmacodynamic interactions of nicotine with its receptors, where continuous exposure to nicotine (e.g., via patch) may lead to receptor desensitization, whereas pulsatile administration allows functional recovery of the receptor and hence further stimulation. As our understanding of cholinergic system evolves, more therapeutic targets for neurodegenerative and/or neuropsychiatric diseases are anticipated.

Acknowledgements

This work was supported in part by NIH/NIAAA R03AA022479; NIH/NIGMS (2S06 GM08016-39) (YT); the National Institute of Health (NIH) R25 Resource Grant (1 R25 AG047843-01) (ABC), the National Science Foundation [NSF IOS-1355034] (TH), Howard University College of Medicine (TH), and the District of Columbia Center for AIDS Research, an NIH funded program [P30AI117970] (TH), which is supported by the following NIH Co-Funding and Participating Institutes and Centers: NIAID, NCI, NICHD, NHLBI, NIDA, NIMH, NIA, NIDDK, NIMHD, NIDCR, NINR, FIC and OAR. The content is solely the responsibility of the authors and does not necessarily represent the official views of the NIH.

Conflict of interest

The authors declare no conflict of interest.

Author details

Yousef Tizabi[1*], Bruk Getachew[1], Vassiliy Tsytsarev[2], Antonei B. Csoka[3], Robert L. Copeland[1] and Thomas Heinbockel[3]

1 Department of Pharmacology, Howard University College of Medicine, Washington, DC, USA

2 School of Medicine, University of Maryland, Baltimore, MD, USA

3 Department of Anatomy, Howard University College of Medicine, Washington, DC, USA

*Address all correspondence to: ytizabi@howard.edu

References

[1] Pasquini J, Brooks DJ, Pavese N. The cholinergic brain in Parkinson's disease. Movement Disorders in Clinical Practice. 2021;**8**(7):1012-1026. DOI: 10.1002/mdc3.13319

[2] Lee HW, Yang SH, Kim JY, Kim H. The role of the medial Habenula cholinergic system in addiction and emotion-associated Behaviors. Frontiers in Psychiatry. 2019;**10**:100. DOI: 10.3389/fpsyt.2019.00100

[3] Jin Z. Muscarine, imidazole, oxazole and thiazole alkaloids. Natural Product Reports. 2016;**33**(11):1268-1317. DOI: 10.1039/c6np00067c

[4] Volpicelli LA, Levey AI. Muscarinic acetylcholine receptor subtypes in cerebral cortex and hippocampus. Progress in Brain Research. 2004;**145**:59-66. DOI: 10.1016/S0079-6123(03)45003-6

[5] Haga T. Molecular properties of muscarinic acetylcholine receptors. Proceedings of the Japan Academy. Series B, Physical and Biological Sciences. 2013;**89**(6):226-256. DOI: 10.2183/pjab.89.226

[6] Shapiro MS, Gomeza J, Hamilton SE, Hille B, Loose MD, Nathanson NM, et al. Identification of subtypes of muscarinic receptors that regulate Ca^{2+} and K^{+} channel activity in sympathetic neurons. Life Sciences. 2001;**68**(22-23):2481-2487. DOI: 10.1016/s0024-3205(01)01042-6

[7] Eglen RM. Overview of muscarinic receptor subtypes. Handbook Experimental Pharmacology. 2012;**208**:3-28. DOI: 10.1007/978-3-642-23274-9_1

[8] Miyakawa T, Yamada M, Duttaroy A, Wess J. Hyperactivity and intact hippocampus-dependent learning in mice lacking the M1 muscarinic acetylcholine receptor. The Journal of Neuroscience. 2001;**21**:5239-5250. DOI: 10.1523/JNEUROSCI.21-14-05239.2001

[9] Shinoe T, Matsui M, Taketo MM, Manabe T. Modulation of synaptic plasticity by physiological activation of M1 muscarinic acetylcholine receptors in the mouse hippocampus. The Journal of Neuroscience. 2005;**25**:11194-11200. DOI: 10.1523/jneurosci.2338-05

[10] Anagnostaras SG, Murphy GG, Hamilton SE, Mitchell SL, Rahnama NP, Nathanson NM, et al. Selective cognitive dysfunction in acetylcholine M1 muscarinic receptor mutant mice. Nature Neuroscience. 2003;**6**(1):51-58. DOI: 10.1038/nn992

[11] Tizabi Y, Getachew B, Copeland RL, Aschner M. Nicotine and the nicotinic cholinergic system in COVID-19. The FEBS Journal. 2020;**287**(17):3656-3663. DOI: 10.1111/febs.15521

[12] Tizabi Y, Getachew B, Aschner M. Novel pharmacotherapies in Parkinson's disease. Neurotoxicity Research. 2021;**39**(4):1381-1390. DOI: 10.1007/s12640-021-00375-5

[13] Tizabi Y., Getachew B., Copeland RL., Moratalla R., Patricio F., Ilhuicamina Daniel Limón ID., Del Bel E., Aschner M. Novel pharmacotherapies for L-DOPA-induced dyskinesia. In: Kostrzewa R.M. (eds) Handbook of Neurotoxicity. Springer, Cham. 2021. p 1-19. doi.org/10.1007/978-3-030-71519-9_218-1

[14] Simon T, Kirk J, Dolezalova N, Guyot M, Panzolini C, Bondue A, et al.

The cholinergic anti-inflammatory pathway inhibits inflammation without lymphocyte relay. Frontiers in Neuroscience. 2023;**17**:1125492. DOI: 10.3389/fnins.2023.1125492

[15] Hu S, Wang Y, Li H. The regulation effect of α7nAChRs and M1AChRs on inflammation and immunity in Sepsis. Mediators of Inflammation. 2021;**2021**:9059601. DOI: 10.1155/2021/9059601

[16] Uwada J, Nakazawa H, Muramatsu I, Masuoka T, Yazawa T. Role of muscarinic acetylcholine receptors in intestinal epithelial homeostasis: Insights for the treatment of inflammatory bowel disease. International Journal of Molecular Sciences. 2023;**24**(7):6508. DOI: 10.3390/ijms24076508

[17] Oenema TA, Kolahian S, Nanninga JE, Rieks D, Hiemstra PS, Zuyderduyn S, et al. Pro-inflammatory mechanisms of muscarinic receptor stimulation in airway smooth muscle. Respiratory Research. 2010;**11**(1):130. DOI: 10.1186/1465-9921-11-130

[18] Fernando JC, Hoskins B, Ho IK. The role of dopamine in behavioral supersensitivity to muscarinic antagonists following cholinesterase inhibition. Life Sciences. 1986;**39**(23):2169-2176. DOI: 10.1016/0024-3205(86)90393-0

[19] Grilli M, Zappettini S, Raiteri L, Marchi M. Nicotinic and muscarinic cholinergic receptors coexist on GABAergic nerve endings in the mouse striatum and interact in modulating GABA release. Neuropharmacology. 2009;**56**(3):610-614. DOI: doi.10.1016/j.neuropharm.2008.10.014

[20] Wang H, Sun X. Desensitized nicotinic receptors in brain. Brain Research. Brain Research Reviews. 2005;**48**(3):420-437. DOI: 10.1016/j.brainresrev.2004.09.003

[21] Fujii S, Jia Y, Yang A, Sumikawa K. Nicotine reverses GABAergic inhibition of long-term potentiation induction in the hippocampal CA1 region. Brain Research. 2000;**863**(1-2):259-265. DOI: 10.1016/S0006-8993(00)02119-3

[22] Vige X, Briley M. Scopolamine induces up-regulation of nicotinic receptors in intact brain but not in nucleus basalis lesioned rats. Neuroscience Letters. 1988;**88**(3):319-324. DOI: 10.1016/0304-3940(88)90231-5

[23] Meyerhoff WL. Surgical section of the posterior ampullary nerve. The Laryngoscope. 1985;**95**(8):933-935. DOI: 10.1288/00005537-198508000-00009

[24] Pulkrabkova L, Svobodova B, Konecny J, Kobrlova T, Muckova L, Janousek J, et al. Neurotoxicity evoked by organophosphates and available countermeasures. Archives of Toxicology. 2023;**97**(1):39-72. DOI: 10.1007/s00204-022-03397-w

[25] Parker JC, Sarkar D, Quick MW, Lester RA. Interactions of atropine with heterologously expressed and native alpha 3 subunit-containing nicotinic acetylcholine receptors. British Journal of Pharmacology. 2003;**138**(5):801-810. DOI: 10.1038/sj.bjp.0705124

[26] Galvin VC, Yang ST, Paspalas CD, Yang Y, Jin LE, Datta D, et al. Muscarinic M1 receptors modulate working memory performance and activity via KCNQ potassium channels in the primate prefrontal cortex. Neuron. 2020;**106**(4):649-661. DOI: 10.1016/j.neuron.2020.02.030

[27] Vijayraghavan S, Everling S. Neuromodulation of persistent activity

and working memory circuitry in primate prefrontal cortex by muscarinic receptors. Frontier in Neural Circuits. 2021;**15**:648624. DOI: 10.3389/fncir.2021.648624

[28] Upright NA, Baxter MG. Effects of nicotinic antagonists on working memory performance in young rhesus monkeys. Neurobiology of Learning and Memory. 2021;**184**:107505. DOI: 10.1016/j.nlm.2021.107505

[29] Sawagashira R, Tanaka M. Nicotine promotes the utility of short-term memory during visual search in macaque monkeys. Psychopharmacology. 2022;**239**(9):3019-3029. DOI: 10.1007/s00213-022-06186-6

[30] Galvin VC, Yang S, Lowet AS, Datta D, Duque A, Arnsten AF, et al. M1 receptors interacting with NMDAR enhance delay-related neuronal firing and improve working memory performance. Current Research Neurobiology. 2021;**2**:100016. DOI: 10.1016/j.crneur.2021.100016

[31] Erskine FF, Ellis JR, Ellis KA, Stuber E, Hogan K, Miller V, et al. Evidence for synergistic modulation of early information processing by nicotinic and muscarinic receptors in humans. Human Psychopharmacology. 2004;**19**(7):503-509. DOI: 10.1002/hup.613

[32] Ellis JR, Ellis KA, Bartholomeusz CF, Harrison BJ, Wesnes KA Erskine FF et al. Muscarinic and nicotinic receptors synergistically modulate working memory and attention in humans, The International Journal of Neuropsychopharmacology 2006; 9(2): 175-189, doi.10.1017/S1461145705005407

[33] Leblond L, Beaufort C, Delerue F, Durkin TP. Differential roles for nicotinic and muscarinic cholinergic receptors in sustained visuo-spatial attention? A study using a 5-arm maze protocol in mice. Behavioural Brain Research. 2002;**128**(1):91-102. DOI: doi.10.1016/S0166-4328(01)00306-0

[34] Green A, Ellis KA, Ellis J, Bartholomeusz CF, Ilic S, Croft RJ, et al. Muscarinic and nicotinic receptor modulation of object and spatial n-back working memory in humans. Pharmacology, Biochemistry, and Behavior. 2005;**81**(3):575-584. DOI: 10.1016/j.pbb.2005.04.010

[35] Feiro O, Thomas J. The interactive effects of nicotinic and muscarinic cholinergic receptor inhibition on fear conditioning in young and aged C57BL/6 mice. Pharmacology Biochemistry and Behavior. 2005;**80**(2):251-262. DOI: 10.1016/j.pbb.2004.11.005

[36] Guizzetti M, Moore NH, Giordano G, Costa LG. Modulation of neuritogenesis by astrocyte muscarinic receptors. The Journal of Biological Chemistry. 2008;**283**(46):31884-31897. DOI: 10.1074/jbc.M801316200

[37] Lee C, Daggett A, Gu XS, Jiang L, Langfelder P, Li X, et al. Elevated TREM2 gene dosage reprograms microglia responsivity and ameliorates pathological phenotypes in Alzheimer's disease models. Neuron. 2018;**97**:1032-1048. DOI: 10.1016/j.neuron.2018.02.002

[38] Wei Y, Li X. Different phenotypes of microglia in animal models of Alzheimer disease. Immunity & Ageing. 2022;**19**:44. DOI: 10.1186/s12979-022-00300-0

[39] Raber J, Caruncho HJ, De Deurwaerdere P, Grilli M. Editorial: Insights on neuroinflammatory response by microglia-targeted pharmacology. Frontiers in Pharmacology. 2023;**14**:1205. DOI: doi.org/10.3389/fphar.2023.1205859

[40] Huang W, Xia Q, Zheng F, Zhao X, Ge F, Xiao J, et al. Microglia-mediated neurovascular unit dysfunction in Alzheimer's disease. Journal of Alzheimer's Disease. 2023. DOI: 10.3233/JAD-221064

[41] Tanzi RE. The genetics of Alzheimer disease. Cold Spring Harbor Perspectives in Medicine. 2012;**2**(10):a006296. DOI: 10.1101/cshperspect.a006296

[42] Morris JC, Weiner M, Xiong C, Beckett L, Coble D, Saito N, et al. Autosomal dominant and sporadic late onset Alzheimer's disease share a common in vivo pathophysiology. Brain. 2022;**145**(10):3594-3607. DOI: 10.1093/brain/awac181

[43] Sobue A, Komine O, Yamanaka K. Neuroinflammation in Alzheimer's disease: Microglial signature and their relevance to disease. Inflammation Regeneration. 2023;**43**(1):26. DOI: 10.1186/s41232-023-00277-3

[44] Valles SL, Singh SK, Campos-Campos J, Colmena C, Campo-Palacio I, Alvarez-Gamez K, et al. Functions of astrocytes under Normal conditions and after a brain disease. International Journal of Molecular Sciences. 2023;**24**(9):8434. DOI: 10.3390/ijms24098434

[45] Qian K, Jiang X, Liu ZQ, Zhang J, Fu P, Su Y, et al. Revisiting the critical roles of reactive astrocytes in neurodegeneration. Molecular Psychiatry. 2023. DOI: 10.1038/s41380-023-02061-8

[46] Fontana IC, Kumar A, Nordberg A. The role of astrocytic α7 nicotinic acetylcholine receptors in Alzheimer disease. Nature Reviews. Neurology. 2023;**19**:278-288. DOI: 10.1038/s41582-023-00792-4

[47] Kim KY, Shin KY, Chang KA. GFAP as a potential biomarker for Alzheimer's disease: A systematic review and Meta-analysis. Cell. 2023;**12**(9):1309. DOI: 10.3390/cells12091309

[48] Díaz-Castro B, Robel S, Mishra A. Astrocyte Endfeet in brain function and pathology: Open questions. Annual Review of Neuroscience. 2023. DOI: 10.1146/annurev-neuro-091922-031205

[49] Yue Q, Xu Y, Lin L, Hoi MPM. Canthin-6-one (CO) from Picrasma quassioides (D.Don) Benn. ameliorates lipopolysaccharide (LPS)-induced astrocyte activation and associated brain endothelial disruption. Phytomedicine. 2022;**101**:154108. DOI: 10.1016/j.phymed.2022.154108

[50] Shen Z, Li ZY, Yu MT, Tan KL, Chen S. Metabolic perspective of astrocyte dysfunction in Alzheimer's disease and type 2 diabetes brains. Biomedicine & Pharmacotherapy. 2023;**158**:114206. DOI: 10.1016/j.biopha.2022.114206

[51] Li L, Liu Z, Jiang YY, Shen WX, Peng YP, Qiu YH. Acetylcholine suppresses microglial inflammatory response via α7nAChR to protect hippocampal neurons. Journal of Integrative Neuroscience. 2019;**18**(1):51-56. DOI: 10.31083/j.jin.2019.01.114

[52] McKee CG, Hoffos M, Vecchiarelli HA, Tremblay MÈ. Microglia: A pharmacological target for the treatment of age-related cognitive decline and Alzheimer's disease. Frontiers in Pharmacology. 2023;**14**:1125982. DOI: 10.3389/fphar.2023.1125982

[53] Chen XF, Al E, Manis M, Herz J, Smirnov I, Aladyeva E, et al. Microglia-mediated T cell infiltration drives

neurodegeneration in tauopathy. Nature. 2023;**615**:668-677. DOI: 10.1038/s41586-023-05788-0

[54] Pannell M, Meier MA, Szulzewsky F, Matyash V, Endres M, Kronenberg G, et al. The subpopulation of microglia expressing functional muscarinic acetylcholine receptors expands in stroke and Alzheimer's disease. Brain Structure & Function. 2016;**221**(2):1157-1172. DOI: 0.1007/s00429-014-0962-y

[55] Wieczorek M, Abualrous ET, Sticht J, Álvaro-Benito M, Stolzenberg S, Noé F, et al. Major histocompatibility complex (MHC) class I and MHC class II proteins: Conformational plasticity in antigen presentation. Frontiers in Immunology. 2017;**8**:292. DOI: 10.3389/fimmu.2017.00292

[56] Li WP, Su XH, Hu NY, Hu J, Li XW, Yang JM, et al. Astrocytes mediate cholinergic regulation of adult hippocampal neurogenesis and memory through M1muscarinic receptor. Biological Psychiatry. 2022;**92**(12):984-998. DOI: 10.1016/j.biopsych.2022.04.019

[57] Khakpai F, Nasehi M, Haeri-Rohani A, Eidi A, Zarrindast MR. Septo-hippocampo-septal loop and memory formation. Basic. Clinical Neuroscience. 2013;**4**(1):5-23

[58] Valentine G, Sofuoglu M. Cognitive effects of nicotine: Recent Progress. Current Neuropharmacology. 2018;**16**(4):403-414. DOI: 10.2174/1570159X15666171103152136

[59] Oleksak P, Novotny M, Patocka J, Nepovimova E, Hort J, Pavlik J, et al. Neuropharmacology of cevimeline and muscarinic drugs-focus on cognition and neurodegeneration. International Journal of Molecular Sciences. 2021;**22**(16):8908. DOI: 10.3390/ijms22168908

[60] Peter J, Mayer I, Kammer T, Minkova L, Lahr J, Klöppel S, et al. The relationship between cholinergic system brain structure and function in healthy adults and patients with mild cognitive impairment. Scientific Reports. 2021;**11**(1):16080. DOI: 10.1038/s41598-021-95573-8

[61] Chen ZR, Huang JB, Yang SL, Hong FF. Role of cholinergic signaling in Alzheimer's disease. Molecules. 2022;**27**(6):1816. DOI: doi.org/10.3390/molecules27061816

[62] Zheng J, Zhu H, Zhao Z, Du M, Wang Z, Lan L, et al. Vesicular acetylcholine transporter in the basal forebrain improves cognitive impairment in chronic cerebral hypoperfusion rats by modulating theta oscillations in the hippocampus. Neuroscience Letters. 2023;**807**:137281. DOI: 10.1016/j.neulet.2023.137281

[63] Aryal SP, Fu X, Sandin JN, Neupane KR, Lakes JE, Grady ME, et al. Nicotine induces morphological and functional changes in astrocytes via nicotinic receptor activity. Glia. 2021;**69**(8):2037-2053. DOI: 10.1002/glia.24011

[64] Brown D, Ramlochansingh C, Manaye KF, Tizabi Y. Nicotine promotes survival of cells expressing amyloid precursor protein and presenilin: Implication for Alzheimer's disease. Neuroscience Letters. 2013;**535**:57-61. DOI: 10.1016/j.neulet.2012.12.046

[65] Tizabi Y. Duality of antidepressants and neuroprotectants. Neurotoxicity Research. 2016;**30**(1):1-13. DOI: 10.1007/s12640-015-9577-1

[66] Tizabi Y, Getachew B. Nicotinic receptor intervention in Parkinson's disease: Future directions. Clinical Pharmacological Translational Medicine. 2017;**1**(1):14-19

[67] van der Zee EA, Streefland C, Strosberg AD, Schröder H, Luiten PGM. Visualization of cholinoceptive neurons in the rat neocortex: Colocalization of muscarinic and nicotinic acetylcholine receptors. Molecular Brain Research. 1992;**14**(4):326-336. DOI: doi.10.1016/0169-328X(92)90100-P

[68] Rehman MU, Sehar N, Dar NJ, Khan A, Arafah A, Rashid S, et al. Mitochondrial dysfunctions, oxidative stress and neuroinflammation as therapeutic targets for neurodegenerative diseases: An update on current advances and impediments. Neuroscience and Biobehavioral Reviews. 2023;**144**:104961

[69] Teleanu DM, Niculescu AG, Lungu II, Radu CI, Vladâcenco O, Roza E, et al. An overview of oxidative stress, Neuroinflammation, and neurodegenerative diseases. International Journal of Molecular Sciences. 2022;**23**(11):5938

[70] Crans RAJ, Ciruela F. Dopaminergic-cholinergic imbalance in movement disorders: A role for the novel striatal dopamine D2- muscarinic acetylcholine M1 receptor heteromer. Neural Regeneration Research. 2021;**16**(7):1406-1408. DOI: 10.4103/1673-5374.300988

[71] Iarkov A, Mendoza C, Echeverria V. Cholinergic receptor modulation as a target for preventing dementia in Parkinson's disease. Frontiers in Neuroscience. 2021;**15**:665820. DOI: 10.3389/fnins.2021.665820

[72] Tikhonova MA, Chang H-M, Singh SK, Vieau D. Editorial: Experimental and innovative approaches to multi-target treatment of Parkinson's and Alzheimer's diseases. Frontiers in Neuroscience. 2022;**16**:910020. DOI: 10.3389/fnins.2022.910020

[73] Di Bari M, Di Pinto G, Reale M, Mengod G, Tata AM. Cholinergic system and Neuroinflammation: Implication in multiple sclerosis. Central Nervous System Agents in Medicinal Chemistry. 2017;**17**(2):109-115. DOI: 10.2174/1871524916666160822115133

[74] Gatta V, Mengod G, Reale M, Tata AM. Possible correlation between cholinergic system alterations and neuro/inflammation in multiple sclerosis. Biomedicine. 2020;**8**(6):153

Chapter 4

Modes of Acetylcholine Signaling in the Prefrontal Cortex: Implications for Cholinergic Dysfunction and Disorders

Matthew Fecik and Lisa M. Savage

Abstract

The forebrain cholinergic system is an important mediator of arousal, attention, memory, and other cognitive processes. Cholinergic signaling is typically divided into two patterns, tonic signaling, which involves sustained changes in ambient acetylcholine (ACh) tone over seconds to minutes, and phasic signaling, which involves fast changing, spatially specific release of ACh on a millisecond timescale. There is evidence to suggest unique functional roles for both types of signaling in the prefrontal cortex: phasic release of ACh is thought to be necessary for attentional processes, as well as cue detection, while tonic signaling is thought to be involved in regulating global arousal states and has been shown to increase with general cognitive demand. The differences between these two types of signaling may originate from electrophysiological properties of cholinergic cell types, distinct muscarinic and nicotinic receptor utilization and/or expression, and/or differential hydrolysis of ACh by acetylcholinesterase. This review will summarize the current views on the functional role of each type of signaling, while the contributions of ACh receptors, hydrolysis, and basal forebrain anatomy are examined. Additionally, the implications of these factors in ACh signaling will be examined in terms of cholinergic circuit dysfunction that occurs in neurodegenerative diseases.

Keywords: acetylcholine, prefrontal cortex, attention, arousal, Alzheimer's disease, alcohol use disorder

1. Introduction

While the role of acetylcholine (ACh) as a neuromodulatory regulator of REM sleep, global arousal states, and consciousness in the prefrontal cortex has been known for quite some time [1–3], the evidence that ACh also functions as a fast-acting neurotransmitter on a precise spatial and temporal scale to carry out specific cognitive operations has only begun to be explored within the past two decades, with progress accelerating significantly in recent years [4–6]. Studies elucidating short-duration phasic cholinergic signaling in the cortex have been made possible by the use of techniques for collecting temporally precise data on ACh *in vivo*, beginning with electrochemical detection [7], and more recently including optogenetics and fiber photometry [8–11]. Such techniques open exciting new possibilities to advance our understanding of cholinergic neurotransmission in the brain, and importantly, our understanding and treatment of brain disorders such as Alzheimer's disease (AD) and alcohol use disorder (AUD).

ACh functions in the prefrontal cortex are based on a variety of factors such as cortical cytoarchitecture, receptor utilization, cholinesterase activity, and basal forebrain anatomy. It is therefore necessary to reevaluate our understanding of the literature on disorders of the basal forebrain through the lens of the tonic/phasic ACh signaling distinction. The goal of this review is to define what is currently known about tonic and phasic ACh signaling in the prefrontal cortex, how the heterogeneity between these two types of signaling may arise, review the differences in receptor utilization these two types of transmission require, evaluate the role of acetylcholinesterase activity in this distinction, and review some of the deficits to each type of transmission that occur in both AD and AUD.

2. Modes of ACh signaling and their roles in behavior

2.1 Tonic ACh signaling

Tonic signaling (sometimes referred to as volume transmission) represents the traditional conceptualization of cholinergic transmission in the central nervous system. In this form of signaling, ACh functions as a slow-acting neuromodulator that exerts its effects on timescales of several seconds to minutes or even hours. Neuromodulatory ACh originating from the basal forebrain has been shown to be involved in functions such as the transition between arousal states, REM sleep, and exploratory behavior [2, 12–15]. Tonic signaling tends to lack both spatial and temporal precision.

Early evidence suggested that "ACh efflux" was not only involved in global arousal states but also directly involved in attentional processes and reward-based learning [16–18]. An early study using *in vivo* microdialysis measured ACh efflux in the medial prefrontal cortex (mPFC) during a 5-choice serial reaction time task (5-CSRTT) and found that in male rats that were well trained on this task, there was increased ACh efflux, an effect that was attenuated in rats not previously trained [19]. Interestingly, they found that ACh efflux was positively correlated with the number of trials completed during the session in which the cue light was illuminated for 5 seconds every trial, compared to 0.5 or 0.25 seconds. The authors contribute that this rise is dependent on the fact that the longer stimulus may elongate the saliency of the food reward and novelty of the task, which has been shown to be dependent on ACh [18, 20]. However, a follow-up study demonstrated that the increase in ACh efflux was due to the performance of the task alone, as rats whose reinforcement was yoked to another subject's performance rather than their own did not show the same increase in ACh efflux, despite also receiving the same pattern of rewards and being exposed to the cue stimuli [21]. Later literature would go on to implicate attentional control of behavior, particularly cue detection, as a cognitive function dependent on phasic ACh signaling, not general ACh tone [9, 22, 23].

Understanding of tonic cholinergic signaling came mostly from studies using *in vivo* microdialysis, in which cholinesterase activity is typically inhibited to ensure a sufficient concentration of ACh for electrochemical detection. This leads to a potential misunderstanding of cholinergic activity in the frontal cortex, with some suggesting that ACh "tone" may even be a methodological artifact [4]. One of the reasons for such a conclusion stems from the seemingly hyperefficient action of AChE, which is the main enzyme involved in the hydrolysis of ACh in the synaptic cleft and therefore the termination of its action. However, it has been shown that a sufficient volume of ACh is able to transiently inhibit AChE [24, 25], leading to further increases in ACh that can potentially spill over into the extracellular fluid and increase cholinergic tone. Such a mechanism would involve a positive feedback loop in which significant quantities of ACh release can inhibit AChE, further increasing the concentration of extracellular ACh. However, this inhibition may be short-lived [24, 25], perhaps on the timescale of milliseconds, and therefore may cause small "pulses" of spillover without hindering fast synaptic phasic signaling at the point of inhibition.

However, the possibility that visual attention tasks require both intact tonic and phasic ACh signaling in the mPFC cannot be ruled out, and it is possible that performance on these tasks requires an alert attentional state governed by tonic signaling, which has been shown to mediate shifts in attention, as well as phasic signaling to encode for specific behavioral epochs and serve as an indicator of cue presentation. Such a mechanism would have been missed by the microdialysis approaches. Thus, the possibility that task performance is reliant on phasic signaling, while behavioral engagement is dependent on the ambient tonic signaling that is perpetually present in the cortex cannot be ruled out and the delineation of the two is a potential area of future research.

2.2 Phasic ACh signaling

Contrasted with tonic ACh signaling, phasic signaling involves much faster time scale circuit-specific release. Phasic signaling is thought to be wired, meaning that it involves the release of ACh from a single cell that innervates a single cortical cell in a highly specific manner [4]. Unlike tonic signaling, it does not involve spillover from the synapse into the extracellular fluid, rather it is constrained to the synapse. This type of signaling occurs on a much faster timescale—likely that of only hundreds of milliseconds. This type of signaling has been implicated in cortical control of attention, specifically cue detection—the cognitive process needed to determine whether a cue that signals a reward is present or not [6].

Based on work using mice, it has been demonstrated that projections originating in the nucleus basalis of Meynert (NbM) and substantia innominata (SI), which form the NbM complex, send their axons to the mPFC and are necessary for cue detection [6]. Particularly, it is thought that these projections are involved in the shift between vigilance and cue detection [6]. This is further demonstrated by the fact that disruption of the mPFC's cholinergic innervation impairs cue detection, while disrupting projections to the other targets of the NbM, such as the motor cortex, yields no effect on this task [23]. Phasic ACh signaling in this circuit is likely the causal mediator of cue detection, as it has been shown that optogenetic stimulation of the NbM during a cue detection task improved performance during cued trials and increased the false alarm rate during non-cued trials, suggesting that millisecond timescale cholinergic signaling originating in the NbM is involved directly in the encoding of the representation of the cue in the prefrontal cortex in mice [9].

In addition, there is evidence to suggest that the basal forebrain is involved in the formation of stimulus associations in mice. Tu et al. [11] found that cholinergic signaling during associative conditioning can affect the strength of the association formed in a time-dependent manner. Although the NbM is commonly cited as the primary source of cholinergic projections to the prelimbic cortex (PrL), and injection of retrograde tracer into the PrL revealed that the greatest source of cholinergic innervation originated in the horizontal diagonal band (HDB). Therefore, Tu et al. [11] targeted the PrL projections originating in the HDB for optogenetic manipulation and found that stimulation during the unconditioned stimulus impaired associative learning while inhibition facilitated it. Furthermore, they found that optogenetic stimulation during the conditioned stimulus did not affect the strength of associative learning, but inhibition lead to impaired learning. This was further accompanied by fiber photometry data that show that the level of excitation of the PrL correlates with the strength of the memory, such that ACh signaling during the unconditioned stimulus strengthened across sessions. These data suggest that phasic signaling is uniquely sensitive to timing, such that the functional role of the cholinergic projections from the HDB to the PrL region involves specifically timed excitation, further lending evidence for the role of ACh in encoding specific stimulus representations [11].

One of the ways that cholinergic signaling can be achieved on this timescale is through the actions of acetylcholinesterase (AChE), which is an incredibly effective hydrolytic enzyme, making the local regulation of AChE as one of the ways in which a degree of heterogeneity is introduced between tonic and phasic ACh signaling. Local expression of AChE may contribute to some of the anatomical heterogeneity between tonic and phasic signaling and makes it likely that phasic signaling would occur, due to its potent catalytic action. However, this has not been investigated thoroughly and represents a future area of inquiry. As cholinesterase activity is likely one of the most important regulators of spatially and temporally restricted ACh signaling in the prefrontal cortex, our understanding of its spatial distribution in the cortex is of paramount importance.

2.3 Tonic vs. phasic signaling: differing viewpoints on the distinction

The presence of such a highly potent catalytic mechanism such as the hydrolysis of ACh by AChE has led some to suggest that tonic ACh signaling in the forebrain is unlikely to affect behavior at all. In this view, the fact that the rate-limiting step of ACh hydrolysis is the diffusion of ACh into the synapse, and not the hydrolytic action of AChE itself, is evidence to suggest that ACh is unlikely to travel distances beyond the synapse and therefore changes in extracellular ACh concentration is unlikely to be a contributor to behavioral events [4]. However, others believe that the tonic/phasic distinction is an oversimplification and that ACh signaling most likely has both fast and slow components that both contribute to behavior. In this view, cholinergic signaling varies as a function of anatomy, receptor subtypes, and ACh hydrolysis—and therefore the concept of ACh tone may still have some functional role in behavior [26].

While the exact middle ground between these two viewpoints is yet to be determined, one study demonstrated both relevant tonic and phasic ACh signaling simultaneously in the PFC and dorsal hippocampus of mice in an attempt to differentiate between their functions. Using electrochemical choline biosensors, Teles-Grilo Ruivo et al. [15] demonstrated that tonic ACh signaling during sleep was highest exclusively during REM sleep that preceded wakefulness. They also demonstrated that tonic signaling was highest as the animal approached a reward in a randomized forced alternation T-maze. Additionally, they found that phasic ACh was associated with the presentation of the reward, with phasic signaling showing response halfwidths significantly shorter than during tonic signaling. Importantly, they demonstrated that both tonic and phasic signaling were highly coordinated between the PFC and the dorsal hippocampus, suggesting that not only does such a distinction in modes of ACh transmission exist in the cortex, but likely can be extended to the hippocampus as well. Should this be the case, the drivers of the distinction are likely to be driven by ubiquitous mechanisms such as cholinesterase activity, or some intrinsic property of basal forebrain anatomy. Ruivo et al. [15] suggest that their results demonstrate that tonic ACh signaling, especially during REM sleep, maybe prepare the mPFC and hippocampus for subsequent alertness and later attentional demands.

Additionally, there is electrophysiological evidence to suggest a dichotomy in cholinergic signaling in the basal forebrain. Unal et al. [27] demonstrated that there are two distinct populations of basal forebrain cholinergic neurons that are distinguished by their electrophysiological properties. Early firing neurons were more excitable, quicker firing, and had more pronounced refractory periods following firing, while later firing neurons were less excitable but more sustained in their ACh release. The authors suggested early firing cells may be involved in phasic signaling and therefore be important for attention, while the late firing cells may be involved in tonic signaling and therefore more important for global arousal states [27]. This suggests that the dichotomy has its roots in electrophysiological correlates.

The above work was later expanded on by Laszlovszky and colleagues [28]. They recorded from cells in mice both *in vivo* and *in vitro* and determined that basal forebrain cholinergic neurons took one of two forms, excitable, burst-firing cells (Burst-BFCN) and less excitable, rhythmic cells (Reg-BFCN). They found Burst-BFCN cells to be more numerous than Reg-BFCN in both the NbM and the horizontal limb of the HDB and consisted of two subtypes, ones with regular inter-spike intervals which they refer to as Burst-BFCN-SB and ones with Poisson-like inter-spike intervals which they refer to as Burst-BFCN-PL. They found that Burst-BFCN cells showed cortical synchronicity and fired bursts of action potentials in response to both reward and punishment during an auditory cue detection task. Reg-BFCN cells, on the other hand, were found to have precise spikes after behavioral outcomes, mainly hits, but not false alarms, correct rejections, or misses. Furthermore, there was distinct anatomical heterogeneity amongst these cell types, with Burst-BFCN found in the anterior basal forebrain and Reg-BFCN cells found in the posterior division [28]. These findings offer a unique viewpoint on the current tonic/phasic debate. They contend that such a divide between tonic and phasic signaling does exist and has anatomical and electrophysiological origins. Such an explanation seems to suggest that tonic ACh signaling has a much greater role in cue detection and cognitive operations than would be suggested by Sarter and Lustig [4].

Recently, basal forebrain cholinergic neurons have also been categorized into neurons that express calbindin-D28K (D28K) protein (ChAT D28K+) and those that do not (ChAT D28K-). The expression of D28K across the basal forebrain nuclei ranges significantly. About 40% of ChAT neurons in the VDB co-stain D28K, relative to 30% in the MS, 16% in the HDB, and less than 2% in the NBM [29]. ChAT+ neurons that also stain for D28K have fewer processes and a lower firing frequency. Interestingly, D28K is a Ca^{2+} binding protein that may function to protect cells from Ca^{2+}-dependent neurodegeneration [29]. This is supported by data that the D28K protein is decreased in cholinergic neurons as a function of aging and in AD [30, 31]. Data support that cholinergic neurons are a heterogeneous population of cells, and understanding the unique profiles of the subpopulations may lead to a better understanding of critical behavioral processes they are involved in.

The location of cholinergic neurons is also a predictor of differential function. Amongst the cholinergic nuclei that project to the cortex, the HDB (rostral BF), and NBM/SI (caudal BF), there is data to support differential function across the anatomical location. Early literature on the NbM to prefrontal cortex circuit suggests a limited degree of axon collateralization between individual projection neurons, which limits the crosstalk between cortical cells and layers [32]. Thus, these circuits seem to be suited for phasic signaling, such that limited collateralization allows for a degree of spatial specificity that is necessary for wired cholinergic transmission in the prefrontal cortex. However, there exists some heterogeneity across species in terms of the projection targets of the NbM, such that its innervation of the prelimbic and infralimbic cortex has been well characterized in mice, but the data seem a bit more nuanced in the case of rats, such that retrograde viral tracing does not show NbM innervation of the prelimbic or infralimbic cortices in this species, rather the HDB is the key region [33]. Likewise, there is data to suggest that the mouse prelimbic cortex receives its primary cholinergic innervation from the HDB as well [11].

Assessing cholinergic activity across the BF anteroposterior axis *via* calcium imaging and ACh-specific fiber photometry, it has been revealed that the more rostral cholinergic neurons (HDB) are responsive to pupil change, which marks arousal state, reward delivery, and reward omission. In contrast, cholinergic activity in the caudal region (NbM/SI) was more responsive to unconditioned cues, delivery of shock, and cues that predicted shock [34]. It is therefore possible that the projections of the NbM/SI to the cortex may be important for salient cue detection and that the projections from the HDB to the prefrontal cortex are more critical for appetitive arousal states.

Cortical receptor location within the architectural layers of the cortex may also play a key role in the outcome of ACh signaling. In addition to the aforementioned factors, evidence for tonic and phasic ACh as distinct behaviorally relevant modes of neurotransmission come from the differential roles and actions of muscarinic and nicotinic ACh receptors within the cortex [31]. There is some evidence to suggest that fast nicotinic ACh receptor (nAChR) mediated signaling is essential for phasic ACh signaling in the cortex while muscarinic ACh receptors (mAChR) are involved in slow changes in ACh concentration such as during tonic signaling. However, such a distinction may not be so cut and dry, as there seems to be a degree of muscarinic activity needed to perform a cue detection task [35], which suggests that muscarinic receptor activity may be needed to regulate global arousal states and "prime" the prefrontal cortex for phasic cholinergic signaling.

3. The contribution of acetylcholine receptors in modulating tonic and phasic activity

3.1 Nicotinic receptors

Nicotinic ACh receptors (nAChR) in the cortex have been shown to be essential for a number of cognitive functions, such a top-down attentional control of behavior and general working memory [36, 37]. Given their fast-acting, ionotropic responses, nAChRs are thought to be involved in phasic ACh signaling. Furthermore, given their selective laminar expression throughout different regions of the cortex, it stands to reason that nAChRs would be selectively expressed in circuits where fast, wired ACh transmission is the norm, and in such a distribution that promotes spatially restrained and functionally heterogeneous responses to ACh signaling from the basal forebrain.

While there is evidence to suggest a role for the utilization of these receptors in phasic signaling, the distinction between the role of nAChR in the two modes of cholinergic neurotransmission seems to be much more nuanced.

Much of the evidence surrounding the role of nAChRs in fast synaptic ACh signaling is electrophysiological. It has been shown that the activation of nAChRs evokes short-latency depolarizing postsynaptic potentials in mouse neocortical pyramidal neurons [38], which has been suggested to function as laminar selectivity relative to muscarinic function. Furthermore, nAChR activation throughout the cortex seems to be layer specific, as Poorthuis et al. [39] showed that nAChR activation leads to inhibition of pyramidal cells in the mPFC in layers II and III, but enhanced excitability of layers V and VI. Interestingly, their data suggest that the response to ACh in this region is dependent on different subunits depending on the layer of the cortex. They demonstrated that pyramidal neurons in layer VI exhibit slow inward currents in the presence of ACh that are absent in β2 subunit deficient mice and were blocked by an antagonist for β2 containing nAChRs and were only occasionally accompanied by α7 mediated currents. Meanwhile, layer V mPFC pyramidal cells showed an attenuated response to ACh in α7 deficient mice as well as following the application of an α7 antagonist, but not in β2 deficient mice, suggesting differential expression of these subunits by layer. They also performed two-photon imaging in cortical pyramidal cells of each layer in β2 and α7 deficient mice and found that nAChR-induced neuronal activation is dependent on the β2 subunit when ACh changes in concentration slowly, suggesting that not only is the β2 subunit utilized during tonic signaling, but also potentially reveals an interesting anatomical phenomena in which layer VI, in which β2 containing nAChRs are most involved in, is involved in tonic signaling, while layer V may not be [39].

The idea that nicotinic receptors are involved in tonic ACh signaling is an interesting one as well, in that it would stand as evidence against the assumption nAChRs mediate phasic signaling exclusively, and that tonic signaling is mostly reliant on muscarinic receptors. In addition to its presumed role in the detection of ambient ACh, β2 subunit deletion has been shown to impair attentional performance in mice [40], suggesting a role of such receptor subtypes in phasic ACh signaling, or at least furthering the idea that attentional performance requires some changes in ambient ACh levels. Interestingly enough, the deletion of this subunit can also upregulate muscarinic receptor excitability to compensate in layer VI of the mPFC, which was also seen following the deletion of the α5 subunit as well [41]. The previously mentioned study by Poorthuis and colleagues [39] notably blocked muscarinic receptors to isolate neuronal responses due to nicotinic activation, meaning that such an increase in excitation was masked, and cholinergic tone that would have been detected primarily by muscarinic receptors may have instead bound to nicotinic receptors in layer VI. An alternative explanation is that such a mechanism may allow for further priming of the cortex to ACh signaling to make up for the reduction caused by subunit deletion, allowing for phasic-dependent cognitive processes to attempt to bounce back even in the presence of less cholinergic signaling.

In addition to the β2 subunit, it seems the α5 nAChR subunit is necessary for attention as well, as deletion of the Chrna5 gene, which encodes for the α5 subunit, impairs attention [42]. It was also demonstrated that the loss of Chrna5 delays cholinergic excitation, such that mPFC layer VI pyramidal cells from Chrna5 deficient mice show attenuated onset kinetics but unaffected response magnitude during optogenetic stimulation of cholinergic afferents *in vitro* and that enhancing nicotinic receptor affinity pharmacologically can actually restore the typical response to optogenetic stimulation [8]. The authors suggest that α5 subunit containing nAChRs in the PFC may be necessary to define a critical window for cue detection, such that a delay to their onset results in the animal being unable to properly integrate detected stimuli *via* corticothalamic connections and ends up missing the cue altogether. Another interesting factor that may play into the α5 subunit's role in phasic ACh signaling in cue detection is its relative rarity, in that its expression is much less prevalent than subunits such as β2 [43], and therefore may be more likely to facilitate spatially constrained wired transmission. However, this is yet to be investigated and represents a considerable gap in our understanding of the role of the α5 subunit in attention.

One further subtype that has been implicated in attention control, and by extension, the role of its dysfunction in cognitive decline, is the α7 nAChR which is composed entirely of α7 subunits. This particular subunit has been highly implicated in the cognitive decline associated with AD [44–46]. It has been shown that an α7 nAChR agonist was sufficient to enhance learning speed but not filter distracting information, which was instead enhanced by an α4/ β2 agonist, with no effect on learning speed [47]. Additionally, it has been shown that performance on the 5-choice continuous performance task, a measure of attention in rodents, was improved following the administration of encenicline, a partial agonist to the α7 nAChR, in poor-performing rats [48]. Due to the fact the dysfunction of α7 has been demonstrated in Alzheimer's disease, it is likely that this particular subtype of receptor is necessary for attentional processes in the cortex, in addition to other processes.

3.2 Muscarinic receptors

Muscarinic ACh receptors (mAChR) are thought to be mediators of tonic acetylcholine signaling, due to their longer duration of action *via* G-protein coupled mechanisms that require second messenger signaling. mAChRs are present in the prefrontal cortex both presynaptically and postsynaptically [49]. Thus, they would seem to be much more suited as receptors of tonic signaling, and likely their longer-lasting duration of action and the fact that a single muscarinic receptor can have amplified second messenger signaling lends itself to the idea that muscarinic receptors are involved in relatively slow timescale changes in ACh concentration in the prefrontal cortex. Similarly, such a mechanism would be suitable for the detection of relatively small concentrations of ACh present in the extracellular fluid during tonic transmission, as opposed to the much larger concentration present at the cholinergic synapse during phasic signaling [26].

However, there may be a degree of specificity as to which muscarinic receptor subtypes are involved in tonic signaling. It has been shown that the G_q-coupled M1 mAChR, but not the M3 or M5, is essential to the response of pyramidal neurons to tonic ACh [35], suggesting a role for only specific G_q-coupled receptors, not all of them. This is interesting, as the location of M1 receptors on the dendritic shaft and spines of cortical pyramidal cells provides a degree of anatomical evidence for volume transmission in the cortex, likely meaning that the M1 receptor's anatomical distribution is what favors it toward the detection of ambient ACh over long distances due to the fact that cholinergic neurons are not known to make axo-axonic synapses [50]. These findings point to a specialized role of muscarinic receptors in detecting global, seconds-scale changes in ACh concentration indicative of perisynaptic signaling and tonic transmission.

As mentioned previously, muscarinic receptor activation may serve to "prime" the cortex for subsequent phasic signaling in such a way that both forms of signaling are necessary for attentional processes to occur. A likely mechanism is *via* increases in cortical pyramidal cell excitability, in which muscarinic receptor activation has been shown to alter *via* the induction of LTD in these cells in the medial prefrontal cortex [51]. This is further supported by findings that mice that are deficient in the inhibitory M2 muscarinic receptor show enhanced attentional performance, despite having impaired object-location learning and spontaneous recognition memory [52], suggesting that while the G_q-coupled muscarinic receptors, such as M1, play an important role in cortical excitability, the activation of G_i-coupled receptors such as M2 may be detrimental to attentional performance. It seems likely that muscarinic receptor activation is needed for cue detection and sustained attentional processes, as a non-specific muscarinic receptor antagonist is sufficient to impair attentional performance on a two-choice visual discrimination task in mice [53]. Likewise, M1 receptor antagonism impairs performance on a divided attention task in rats, unlike antagonism of the M4 receptor which did not [54]. Additionally, the M1-positive allosteric modulator TAK-071 has been shown to rescue attentional performance in rats with basal forebrain cholinergic cell loss [55]. Such studies suggest that while muscarinic receptors may play a role in attentional processes, their role in phasic ACh signaling remains unclear.

While it seems that muscarinic receptors are needed for attentional processes due to their effects on global arousal states, the dichotomy of tonic signaling being dependent solely on muscarinic receptors while phasic signaling is dependent solely on nicotinic receptors is evidently an oversimplification. Likely, the mechanism by which attentional control occurs is reliant on both nAChRs and mAChRs, such that mAChRs are needed to orient the organism toward the object of their attention, while nAChRs, at least the α7 and α5 subtypes, are involved in the response of cortical neurons to short timescale phasic ACh release. Thus, both nAChRs and mAChRs seem necessary for phasic ACh signaling and its reliant cognitive operations such as cue detection. However, mAChRs on their own may be mediators of tonic ACh signaling, and thus a degree of tonic ACh efflux is needed to ready the prefrontal cortex for an orientation toward a specific stimulus. However, more research is needed to delineate the contributions of each receptor system to tonic and phasic signaling in the prefrontal cortex, though the way to do so does not seem immediately straightforward.

4. The role of acetylcholinesterase in tonic and phasic ACh signaling

One of the ways in which tonic and phasic ACh signaling are regulated is through the actions of AChE, the catalytic enzyme which hydrolyzes ACh and is thought to be the main determinant of the duration of cholinergic signaling. As stated before, AChE can hydrolyze ACh nearly as fast as the cell can release it, and thus the high catalytic activity of this enzyme is evidence itself of the presence of phasic ACh signaling in the prefrontal cortex. However, it has also been hypothesized that this is one of the reasons as to why tonic ACh signaling is unlikely to directly contribute to behavior at all. Sarter and Lustig [4] state that the fact that AChE is such an efficient hydrolyzer of ACh makes it unlikely for synaptic spillover to occur, and therefore tonic ACh as measured by *in vivo* microdialysis may be a methodological artifact due to the cholinesterase inhibitors perfused into the brain during the process. However, it has been shown that inhibition of AChE by an excess of ACh may occur *via* the formation of a ternary complex [25], which represents one mechanism by which high-ACh concentration can overwhelm AChE and spill over into the extracellular fluid. Therefore, a central role of potentially heterogeneous utilization of AChE during tonic and phasic ACh signaling distinction must be considered.

In the brain, AChE is exclusively expressed as the tailed $AChE_T$ variant. This subunit is able to form an amphiphilic tetramer known as G_4 AChE, which is facilitated by and tethered to proline-rich membrane anchor (PRiMA), anchoring AChE to the presynaptic membrane [56, 57]. Acetylcholinesterase is co-expressed with markers of cholinergic neurons such as choline acetyltransferase (ChAT) *in vivo* [57], suggesting that AChE is likely expressed in cholinergic cells before undergoing tetramerization *via* PRiMA in the endoplasmic reticulum and being transported down the axon [58]. PRiMA likely links tailed G_4 AChE to the presynaptic membrane *via* membrane rafts [59]. Interestingly, PRiMA shows robust co-expression with M1 muscarinic receptors, which are located postsynaptically, suggesting that AChE may originate primarily from cholinergic axons but also intrinsically from neurons in the cortex [60]. Additionally, this co-expression may have interesting functional implications, however, it may simply be due to the ubiquity of expression of the M1 receptor in basal forebrain target regions. To date, no studies have looked to colocalize PRiMA with nicotinic receptors, making any potential differences in PRiMA receptors between neurons expressing the two receptor types is unknown but represents a future area of inquiry.

Experimental manipulations to inhibit the endogenous action of AChE have been shown to cause attentional impairments, such as during a five-choice serial reaction time task in healthy rats [61], suggesting that inhibition of AChE in healthy subjects impairs behaviors likely dependent on phasic signaling. AChE knockout mice have been shown to exhibit a variety of motor deficits due to the role of peripheral AChE in muscle contraction and thermoregulation [62]. Farar et al. [63] characterized PRiMA KO mice on a number of motor and behavioral measures. They found that despite only very subtle motor impairments on the rotarod test and the wire task, these mice had a nearly 200–300-fold increase in extracellular ACh concentration in the striatum as measured *via in vivo* microdialysis during anesthesia, with none of the thermoregulatory impairments seen in mice with a traditional AChE knockout. Additionally, these mice were not impaired on the Morris water maze. Interestingly, they found that the M1 muscarinic receptor was heavily downregulated across all areas of the brain measured, including by approximately 40% in the cortex, with no such decrease in the α7 nAChR or β2-containing nAChRs. One interpretation of these results laid out by the authors is that these data serve as evidence for the hypothesis that AChE is primarily involved in regulating the extracellular ACh concentration, not terminating synaptic transmission [63].

Should that be the case, then it is possible that PRiMA knockout mice may have deficits in phasic ACh signaling, but not tonic signaling. Thus, the hypothesis may be the inverse of what was proposed by these authors, that AChE is primarily utilized at the cholinergic synapses of the prefrontal cortex to rapidly terminate ACh signaling, while ACh "tone" represents ACh that escapes this mechanism and is, therefore, less active during this form of signaling. This may represent a potential mechanism by which attentional and other cognitive impairments occur in disease states that alter AChE and disrupt the balance between ACh release and hydrolysis, such as Alzheimer's disease, while leaving other functions that are dependent on tonic signaling unimpaired until later in the disease.

A likely mechanism for which AChE is inhibited at the synapse, as represented in **Figure 1** is as such: an overabundance of ACh in the synaptic cleft during phasic signaling may lead to inhibition of AChE which allows acetylcholine to spill out of

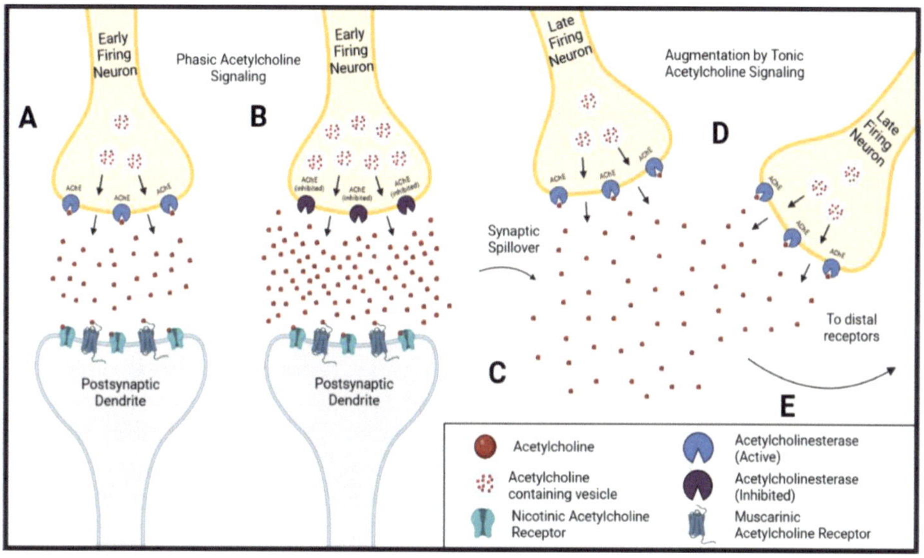

Figure 1.
*Proposed mechanism of the regulation of phasic and tonic acetylcholine (ACh) signaling in the prefrontal cortex. A. Phasic acetylcholine signaling by the terminals of early firing basal forebrain neurons at cholinergic synapses leads to the activation of both postsynaptic nicotinic and muscarinic receptors. The termination of cholinergic signaling is mediated by presynaptic membrane-bound acetylcholinesterase (AChE), which hydrolyzes ACh. B. High levels of phasic firing, such as during high attentional demand, lead to an abundance of ACh at the synapse, inhibiting AChE activity and further increasing the concentration of ACh. C. Synaptic spillover of ACh into the extracellular fluid occurs due to transient inhibition of AChE. D. There is also the release of ACh from the terminals of late-firing basal forebrain cholinergic neurons, which further increases ACh tone. Extracellular ACh is still hydrolyzed by membrane-bound AChE. E. Extracellular ACh travels to distal muscarinic and nicotinic receptors within the prefrontal cortex, modulating global arousal states. *created with BioRender.com*

the synapse and into the extracellular fluid. This ambient ACh would still be under the regulation of AChE, but the enzyme's location on the synaptic membrane would make it more difficult for extracellular acetylcholine to be hydrolyzed, allowing it to accumulate in the extracellular space. Therefore, AChE still regulates ACh tone, albeit mostly indirectly, through its regulation of phasic ACh signaling. Tonic ACh may also be released by non-synaptic terminals, perhaps by specialized basal forebrain cholinergic cells [27, 28], and it is the combination of these two mechanisms that are responsible for ambient ACh fluctuations.

5. ACh in brain disorders: circuit dysfunction

Reductions in markers for the cholinergic phenotype, such as the expression of ChAT, the enzyme necessary for ACh synthesis, are present throughout the basal forebrain following both AD and AUD, a consequence that is considered one of the hallmarks of both of these disorders in particular. These cholinergic deficits are present in two of the main basal forebrain circuits, the projections from the NbM complex (NbM, HDB, SI) to the cortical mantle, and the projections from the MS/DB to the hippocampus. In both disorders, there is a suppression in the basal forebrain cholinergic phenotype. In the case of AUD, there is evidence from animal models to suggest that these deficits may not be permanent and can be rescued *via* the use of voluntary wheel running exercise [64], the actions of neurotrophins [65], and the

AChE inhibitor galantamine [66]. In contrast, chronic treadmill exercise or voluntary wheel running has been shown to attenuate age-related reduction of cholinergic fibers in the cortex and hippocampus and improve some learning and memory outcomes but has minor effects on the number of ChAT [47] positive neurons [67–69]. However, exercise has been shown to improve ACh levels in the hippocampus in an Aβ1–42 peptide rat model [70]. This does suggest that deficits caused by both alcohol-related brain damage and AD may involve a reduction in functional cholinergic neurons, leading to reductions in overall ACh signaling, which can be rescued. It, therefore, seems likely that in both of these disorders there would be a disruption in either, or both, tonic and phasic ACh signaling in the brain.

The drivers of the selective neuropathological vulnerability of cholinergic neurons, across brain disorders, are their large size and extensive projections, which require high metabolic expenditures and trophic factors to maintain the considerable cytoskeletal surface, as well as the machinery for axonal transport over long distances. These morphological properties of cholinergic neurons increase their vulnerability to oxidative stress, neuroinflammation, and altered energy homeostasis that occurs during aging and disease states [71, 72].

Human clinical data have long supported the role of chronic heavy alcohol use leading to premature brain aging, as well as a risk for the development of dementia, including AD [73–77]. Furthermore, alcohol consumption has been linked to an increased risk of dementia in individuals with a genetic predisposition to AD [78, 79]. Recent data from preclinical studies demonstrate that the consequences of adult or developmental EtOH exposure resemble advanced brain aging or produces accelerated AD-related pathology in transgenic models with AD-related transgenes [80–83]. Advanced aging, AD, and AUD have some overlapping neuropathological sequelae: upregulation of proinflammatory markers, suppressed hippocampal neurogenesis, suppression of basal forebrain cholinergic phenotype, and altered pro- and mature NT levels—as well as a change in the ratio of Trk to $p75^{NTRs}$ [84–88]. A common pathway for cholinergic dysfunction in AD and AUD is the disruption of neurotrophins and their receptors (see **Figure 2**), which may drive additive effects of AD and AUD pathology.

5.1 Alzheimer's disease and cholinergic dysfunction

The increase in AChE activity in AD has been known for some time, as many of the drugs currently available for the treatment of this disease target this enzyme and inhibit its activity [89–91]. Cholinesterase inhibition has been shown to increase cognitive performance on the Stroop task in human patients with AD, with the degree of inhibition directly correlating with performance [92]. In AD, AChE inhibitors prolong ACh action, as well as increase the uptake of NGF to improve cholinergic neuronal survival [93]. Furthermore, cholinesterase inhibitor therapy in AD improves cognitive performance by increasing the activation of frontal cortical circuits as determined by fMRI studies [94, 95]. However, only a subset of patients with AD is effectively responsive to AChE inhibitors, and cholinergic basal forebrain integrity is a key predictor of treatment success [96].

As mentioned previously, it is likely that AChE is needed for both tonic and phasic ACh signaling, but is a more immediate causal effector of phasic signaling. It is likely that tonic signaling is required to ready the cortex for phasic signaling, and AChE inhibition may also work to increase ACh tone and facilitate cognitive performance. However, there may be a degree of specificity for phasic signaling when it comes to this modulation. Should the hypothesis that phasic signaling is more immediately

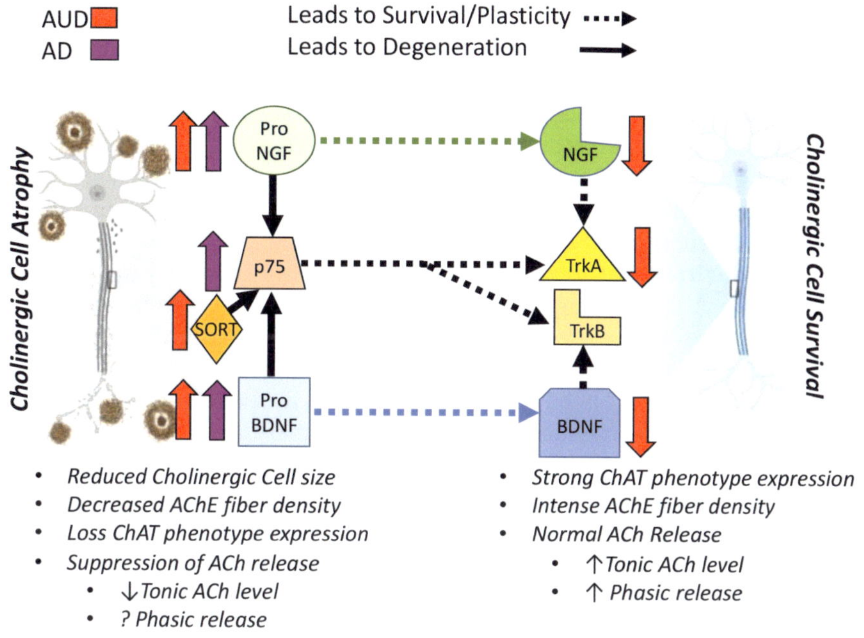

Figure 2.
*Changes in neurotrophins and their receptors that modulate cholinergic cell survival. Both Alzheimer's disease (AD) and alcohol use disorder (AUD) alter the expression and ratio of pro-to-mature nerve growth factor (NGF) and brain-derived growth factor (BDNF), as well as the tropomyosin kinase receptors for NGF (TrkA), BDNF (TrkB), and p75 receptor. The pro-forms of neurotrophins are potent ligands for p75NTR and can induce cell death or loss of cholinergic phenotype when coupled with sortilin. Thus, AUD likely accelerates the pathological sequela of AD. *Created with BioRender.com*

dependent on AChE than tonic signaling be supported, then modulation of AChE should have more of an effect on phasic-dependent processes. However, since tonic signaling is likely needed to modulate phasic signaling and *vice versa*, disentangling these two may be difficult experimentally, since the effects that AChE inhibition may have on tonic signaling may occur after that of phasic signaling, but still on a relatively short pharmacological timescale.

Likely, a balance between ACh and AChE may be critical to the phasic ACh signaling needed for sustained attention. Thus, disorders such as AD disrupt attentional processes by dysregulation of AChE, leading to dysfunction of phasic ACh signaling in the cortex. It has been shown that presenilin-1 (PS1), the catalytic component of the γ secretase complex and therefore the formation of amyloid β (Aβ) [97, 98] affects the processing of PRiMA, as was shown by the use of using hamster ovarian cells transfected with $AChE_T$ and a PS1 conditional knockout mouse. They showed that γ secretase inhibition led to an increase in both PRiMA and $AChE_T$ and that G4 AChE was increased in the membrane rafts in the PFC of PS1 KO mice, representing a potential mechanism by which AD pathology imparts alterations to AChE function [99]. Furthermore, PS1 transgenic mice show increased AChE activity throughout the entirety of the basal forebrain, prior to any behavioral deficits, suggesting that AChE dysfunction may be one of the first steps in the cascade of pathology associated with AD [100]. This increase in AChE activity is typically the therapeutic target of cholinesterase-inhibiting drugs such as donepezil, one of the most widely used drugs for the treatment of AD.

Romberg et al. [101] tested 3xTgAD mice, a strain with APPswe, PS1M146V, and tauP301L mutations to recapitulate some of the major features of AD in humans, on a 5-choice serial reaction time task (5-CSRTT) and found that while the transgenic mice were able to match wild-type controls in performance early on in the task, they would later begin to show impairments across the duration of the task, specifically as stimulus duration was reduced, signifying deficits in sustaining attention. These deficits were rescued *via* the administration of donepezil, demonstrating that inhibiting the alterations to typical AChE activity was sufficient to restore similar functioning to wild-type mice, suggesting that this particular task is reliant on AChE to modulate cortical cholinergic activity [101]. It is likely that AD, through its upregulation of AChE activity, perturbs the frontocortical circuitry necessary for attention by disrupting phasic ACh signaling. Similarly, donepezil was able to reduce scopolamine-induced omissions during the 5-CSRTT, demonstrating that inhibiting AChE can compensate for muscarinic receptor antagonism during this task [102].

Nicotinic receptors have been heavily implicated in the pathogenesis of AD, which likely disrupts nicotinic-dependent signaling in the cortex, and as discussed above has been linked to phasic signaling. This dysfunction likely originates with the SK family of Ca^{2+} sensitive K^{+} channels, as treatment with a selective agonist of these channels improves the nAChR function [103]. Dysfunction with such circuitry is evident by the fact that impairments in sustained attention have been shown using a mouse model of AD [104], demonstrating likely deficits with phasic cholinergic deficits, which, as mentioned before, is at least partially dependent on the utilization of nAChRs in the prefrontal cortex [42, 48]. Additionally, there is some evidence to suggest a link between Aβ pathology and nicotinic dysfunction, as it has been shown that Aβ prevents nicotine-induced inhibitory signaling, but not excitatory signaling, in PFC pyramidal neurons *in vitro* [105], suggesting that Alzheimer's disease pathology may be disrupting the balance of excitation and inhibition necessary for phasic ACh signaling in the PFC. The link between Aβ and nAChR function is further supported by data showing that infusion of Aβ increased α-bungarotoxin autoradiography binding to the α7 nAChR in the frontal cortex exclusively in animals that received weekly attentional stimulation, suggesting that α7 nAChR functionality may be impaired by Aβ, but regular activation of attentional circuitry can activate compensational mechanisms in both the cortex to attempt to restore regular functioning [106].

Similarly, within the cortex itself, there are deficits to muscarinic receptors as well, as M1 mAChR's are being considered as a potential target for treatment [107]. However, work using radioligand labeling of human participants with AD has demonstrated no changes in M1 labeling in the cortex in AD, only in the dentate gyrus [108]. It is possible that despite no changes in M1 expression in the cortex, there are still deficits to its typical function, as postmortem analysis of the brains of individuals with AD showed reduced G-protein coupling of the M1 receptor in the cortex, despite no change in its density [109], mirroring the radioligand results from Scarr et al. [108]. It is possible that impaired function of the M1 receptor in AD serves as an indicator of dysfunctional tonic ACh signaling in the cortex, but as mentioned previously, the relationship between muscarinic receptors and tonic signaling is not one-to-one, and there is likely some contribution of nicotinic receptors to tonic signaling dependent behaviors as well.

5.2 Alcohol use disorder and cholinergic dysfunction

The cholinergic pathology in AUD is similar to that of AD, with some overlap in the effects of binge ethanol exposure during adolescence and age-related cognitive decline [110]. It is therefore likely that alcohol-related damage to the basal forebrain leads to dysfunction of tonic and phasic ACh signaling as well. Acute ethanol exposure in rats has been shown to lead to deficits in sustained attention, demonstrating that phasic ACh signaling in the cortex is likely dysregulated during intoxication [111], though the impairments due to acute ethanol likely have to do with the depressive effect of ethanol throughout the entirety of the brain. However, exposure to binge levels of ethanol in adolescence has been shown to lead to deficits that persist across the lifespan [112–114]. Adolescent intermittent ethanol (AIE) exposure has been shown to lead to reductions in ChAT immunostaining in the NbM in adulthood, an effect exclusive to rats that are exposed to ethanol in adolescence, but not adulthood [115]. This loss of ChAT has been shown to be rescued by galantamine, an AChE inhibitor [66]. Likely, this type of alcohol exposure leads to an upregulation of cholinesterase activity, leading to overactive hydrolysis of ACh that is making it difficult for precisely time-locked phasic ACh signaling to occur, similar to AD.

However, there is some evidence to suggest that overactive AChE is leading to some of these deficits in ways beyond its disruption of phasic ACh signaling. It has been shown that overactive AChE induces apoptosis in both living mice and cell cultures exposed to ethanol [116], suggesting that it is possible that ethanol may overstimulate AChE activity and lead to an apoptotic cascade. However, it is unclear how this relates to the rescue of alcohol-related deficits to cholinergic phenotype, as it has been shown that ChAT cells in the basal forebrain are not dead following exposure to binge levels of ethanol in adolescence, but rather are entering a quiescent state that can be rescued either *via* neurotrophins [65], cholinesterase inhibiting drugs [66], or voluntary wheel running exercise [64]. The relation between the quiescent state these cells take, and the apoptotic mechanism described is yet to be ascertained.

Similarly, AIE has been shown to have effects on tonic ACh signaling in the prefrontal cortex. Adolescent alcohol exposure has been shown to attenuate behaviorally relevant acetylcholine efflux in the PFC during a spontaneous alternation task, which was accompanied by reductions in ChAT in the NbM and the medial septum/diagonal band (MS/DB), suggesting that AIE disrupts innervation of the PFC by the basal forebrain, leading to a reduction in cholinergic tone [117]. Likely, ACh tone is needed during this task to induce a state of general arousal in which the animal is actively attenuating to extra-maze cues to determine the arms of the maze it has visited already and to avoid visiting the same arms consecutively [13]. Fernandez and Savage [112] also demonstrated parallel behavioral impairments, as rats exposed to AIE showed deficits on operant attention set-shifting task, a task that has been shown to be dependent on the mPFC [118]. The exact role of phasic ACh signaling during this task is yet to be investigated, but it is possible that the detection of a visual cue to indicate which of the two levers indicates reward is dependent on a similar mechanism to cue detection in the sustained attention task, and the fact that AIE rats are impaired on the shift from spatial side reinforcement to a visual cue determining reinforcement suggests that these two tasks may be dependent on similar mechanisms. However, more work is needed to determine whether phasic acetylcholine signaling is required for attention.

Other models of alcohol-related brain damage have shown similar effects on the cholinergic system and the prefrontal cortex. For example, adult rats either fed a pyrithiamine deficient diet (PTD), given access to ethanol in their drinking bottles (CET), or a combination of both (PTD-CET) were shown to have impaired spontaneous alternation behavior and reduced ACh efflux in the mPFC during this task, which was accompanied by a reduced latency to lever press during a set shift during operant attention set shifting despite no impairment in performance [119]. This suggests that there are tonic ACh signaling deficits in this model, as demonstrated by the decreased ACh efflux, as well as possible phasic signaling deficits, as the increased amount of time needed to make a lever press in PTD, CET, and PTD-CET animals suggests that the time course of ACh signaling in PFC is being disrupted. The deficits seen during spontaneous alternation during PTD have been shown to be rescued by the AChE inhibitor tacrine [120], suggesting a role of AChE overexpression in the pathology seen in this disorder, suggesting that overactive AChE, mirroring what is seen in AD, is responsible for the tonic ACh deficits. Presumably, these deficits would extend to phasic ACh-dependent processes, but they were not tested here. The fact that cholinesterase inhibition has such an effect on tonic signaling is interesting, but not surprising, as while the mechanism proposed within this review suggests that AChE is more important for phasic signaling, it is nevertheless required to regulate ACh tone as well, exerting its actions both directly by hydrolyzing extracellular ACh and indirectly by regulating phasic signaling and synaptic spillover.

Alcohol-related brain damage and AD seem to converge on the cholinergic system, and the projections from the basal forebrain to the prefrontal cortex seem to be a set of circuits that show particular vulnerability to perturbations. Dysfunction of these circuits likely has effects on both tonic and phasic ACh signaling simultaneously, and it seems that, at the moment, it would be conceptually difficult to investigate an experimental manipulation that would affect one type of signaling but not the other. However, it may be possible to determine whether the time course of the impairments seen in these two types of signaling differ, such that perhaps phasic signaling is first affected by the early cholinergic deficits seen in AD, which later expands to tonic signaling deficits later on. This remains to be determined and represents a future direction for research into modes of ACh signaling.

6. Conclusions and future directions

As the distinction between the roles of tonic and phasic ACh signaling becomes clearer, it is important to understand the specific dysfunction that is occurring in both of these types of signaling in the cortex in disorders such as AD and AUD. It is likely that these two disorders have effects on both muscarinic and nicotinic ACh receptors and that these deficits are part of what is driving the dysregulation of the two types of ACh signaling in the cortex. Additionally, the role of AChE in this distinction cannot be overstated, as its role in hydrolyzing synaptic ACh may be one of the most important regulators of phasic ACh, with its inhibition by high ACh concentrations possibly leading to spillover into the extracellular space and therefore augmenting ACh tone that is usually otherwise due to a different set of basal forebrain cholinergic cells.

The availability of fluorescent ACh sensors for fiber photometry allows for the measurement of ACh activity in vivo on a second timescale. Studies in which changes to ACh signaling following alterations to normal AChE activity can be assessed and are needed to determine the exact role of this enzyme in cortical cholinergic synapses, and how its dysfunction relates to some of the deficits seen in common cholinergic disorders. Likewise, the contribution of alterations to typical nAChR and mAChR function in the PFC to phasic ACh signaling could be investigated using photometric methods. Studies looking directly into how tonic and phasic ACh utilize different cellular machinery seem to be elusive for now, but further breakthroughs in the field could lead to new avenues to address this gap in the literature.

Furthermore, reexamining AD and alcohol-related brain damage through the lens of the tonic phasic distinction may allow researchers to hone in on the exact mechanisms by which cholinergic dysfunction occurs in these diseases and therefore develop new treatments. A reconceptualization of these disorders in terms of the mounting evidence that ACh in the prefrontal cortex is phasic in regard to many of the cognitive symptoms seen in AD may lead us to a better understanding of how the current pharmacological treatments for these diseases work and how to improve them. Similarly, updating our understanding of alcohol-related brain damage using this new conceptualization of ACh signaling in the prefrontal cortex may lead the field into novel treatments and ways to prevent or even reverse cholinergic deficits that arise *via* exposure to heavy amounts of alcohol. Such advancements may be possible with a reevaluation of the way that ACh signaling in the cortex contributes to behavior.

Author details

Matthew Fecik and Lisa M. Savage*
Program in Behavioral Neuroscience, Department of Psychology, Binghamton University, Binghamton, NY, USA

*Address all correspondence to: lsavage@binghamton.edu

References

[1] Jones BE. Arousal and sleep circuits. Neuropsychopharmacology. 2020;**45**(1):6-20. DOI: 10.1038/s41386-019-0444-2

[2] Poulet JFA, Crochet S. The cortical states of wakefulness. Frontiers in Systems Neuroscience. 2018;**12**:64. DOI: 10.3389/fnsys.2018.00064

[3] Perry E, Walker M, Grace J, Perry R. Acetylcholine in mind: A neurotransmitter correlate of consciousness? Trends in Neurosciences. 1999;**22**(6):273-280. DOI: 10.1016/s0166-2236(98)01361-7

[4] Sarter M, Lustig C. Forebrain cholinergic signaling: Wired and phasic, not tonic, and causing behavior. The Journal of Neuroscience. 2020;**40**(4):712-719. DOI: 10.1523/JNEUROSCI.1305-19.2019

[5] Parikh V, Bangasser DA. Cholinergic Signaling dynamics and cognitive control of attention. Current Topics in Behavioral Neurosciences. 2020;**45**:71-87. DOI: 10.1007/7854_2020_133

[6] Sarter M, Lustig C, Berry AS, Gritton H, Howe WM, Parikh V. What do phasic cholinergic signals do? Neurobiology of Learning and Memory. 2016;**130**:135-141. DOI: 10.1016/j.nlm.2016.02.008

[7] Bruno JP, Gash C, Martin B, Zmarowski A, Pomerleau F, Burmeister J, et al. Second-by-second measurement of acetylcholine release in prefrontal cortex. The European Journal of Neuroscience. 2006;**24**(10):2749-2757. DOI: 10.1111/j.1460-9568.2006.05176.x

[8] Venkatesan S, Lambe EK. Chrna5 is essential for a rapid and protected response to Optogenetic release of endogenous acetylcholine in prefrontal cortex. The Journal of Neuroscience. 2020;**40**(38):7255-7268. DOI: 10.1523/JNEUROSCI.1128-20.2020

[9] Gritton HJ, Howe WM, Mallory CS, Hetrick VL, Berke JD, Sarter M. Cortical cholinergic signaling controls the detection of cues. Proceedings of the National Academy of Sciences of the United States of America. 2016;**113**(8):E1089-E1097. DOI: 10.1073/pnas.1516134113

[10] Jing M, Li Y, Zeng J, Huang P, Skirzewski M, Kljakic O. et al. An optimized acetylcholine sensor for monitoring in vivo cholinergic activity. Nature Methods. 2020;17(11): 1139-1146. DOI: 10.1038/ s41592-020-0953-2

[11] Tu G, Halawa A, Yu X, Gillman S, Takehara-Nishiuchi K. Outcome-locked cholinergic Signaling suppresses prefrontal encoding of stimulus associations. The Journal of Neuroscience. 2022;**42**(20):4202-4214. DOI: 10.1523/JNEUROSCI.1969-21.2022

[12] Giovannini MG, Bartolini L, Kopf SR, Pepeu G. Acetylcholine release from the frontal cortex during exploratory activity. Brain Research. 1998;**784**(1-2):218-227. DOI: 10.1016/s0006-8993(97)01161-x

[13] Lalonde R. The neurobiological basis of spontaneous alternation. Neuroscience and Biobehavioral Reviews. 2002;**26**(1):91-104. DOI: 10.1016/s0149-7634(01)00041-0

[14] Sarter M, Bruno JP. Cortical cholinergic inputs mediating arousal, attentional processing and dreaming: Differential afferent regulation of the basal forebrain by telencephalic and brainstem afferents. Neuroscience.

2000;**95**(4):933-952. DOI: 10.1016/s0306-4522(99)00487-x

[15] Teles-Grilo Ruivo LM, Baker KL, Conway MW, Kinsley PJ, Gilmour G, Phillips KG, et al. Coordinated acetylcholine release in prefrontal cortex and Hippocampus is associated with arousal and reward on distinct timescales. Cell Reports. 2017;**18**(4):905-917. DOI: 10.1016/j.celrep.2016.12.085

[16] Himmelheber AM, Sarter M, Bruno JP. Operant performance and cortical acetylcholine release: Role of response rate, reward density, and non-contingent stimuli. Brain Research. Cognitive Brain Research. 1997;**6**(1):23-36. DOI: 10.1016/s0926-6410(97)00014-1

[17] Himmelheber AM, Sarter M, Bruno JP. Increases in cortical acetylcholine release during sustained attention performance in rats. Brain Research. Cognitive Brain Research. 2000;**9**(3):313-325. DOI: 10.1016/s0926-6410(00)00012-4

[18] Inglis FM, Fibiger HC. Increases in hippocampal and frontal cortical acetylcholine release associated with presentation of sensory stimuli. Neuroscience. 1995;**66**(1):81-86. DOI: 10.1016/0306-4522(94)00578-s

[19] Passetti F, Dalley JW, O'Connell MT, Everitt BJ, Robbins TW. Increased acetylcholine release in the rat medial prefrontal cortex during performance of a visual attentional task. The European Journal of Neuroscience. 2000;**12**(8):3051-3058. DOI: 10.1046/j.1460-9568.2000.00183.x

[20] Acquas E, Wilson C, Fibiger HC. Conditioned and unconditioned stimuli increase frontal cortical and hippocampal acetylcholine release: Effects of novelty, habituation, and fear. The Journal of Neuroscience. 1996;**16**(9):3089-3096 https://www.ncbi.nlm.nih.gov/pubmed/8622138

[21] Dalley JW, McGaughy J, O'Connell MT, Cardinal RN, Levita L, Robbins TW. Distinct changes in cortical acetylcholine and noradrenaline efflux during contingent and noncontingent performance of a visual attentional task. The Journal of Neuroscience. 2001;**21**(13):4908-4914 https://www.ncbi.nlm.nih.gov/pubmed/11425918

[22] Sarter M, Lustig C. Cholinergic double duty: Cue detection and attentional control. Current Opinion in Psychology. 2019;**29**:102-107. DOI: 10.1016/j.copsyc.2018.12.026

[23] Parikh V, Kozak R, Martinez V, Sarter M. Prefrontal acetylcholine release controls cue detection on multiple timescales. Neuron. 2007;**56**(1):141-154. DOI: 10.1016/j.neuron.2007.08.025

[24] Massoulie J, Pezzementi L, Bon S, Krejci E, Vallette FM. Molecular and cellular biology of cholinesterases. Progress in Neurobiology. 1993;**41**(1):31-91. DOI: 10.1016/0301-0082(93)90040-y

[25] Hofer P, Fringeli UP. Acetylcholinesterase kinetics. Biophysical Structure Mechanism. 1981;**8**(1-2):45-59. DOI: 10.1007/BF01047105

[26] Disney AA, Higley MJ. Diverse spatiotemporal scales of cholinergic signaling in the neocortex. The Journal of Neuroscience. 2020;**40**(4):720-725. DOI: 10.1523/JNEUROSCI.1306-19.2019

[27] Unal CT, Golowasch JP, Zaborszky L. Adult mouse basal forebrain harbors two distinct cholinergic populations defined by their electrophysiology. Frontiers in Behavioral Neuroscience. 2012;**6**:21. DOI: 10.3389/fnbeh.2012.00021

[28] Laszlovszky T, Schlingloff D, Hegedus P, Freund TF, Gulyas A, Kepecs A, et al. Distinct synchronization, cortical coupling and behavioral function of two basal forebrain cholinergic neuron types. Nature Neuroscience. 2020;**23**(8):992-1003. DOI: 10.1038/s41593-020-0648-0

[29] Li X, Yu H, Zhang B, Li L, Chen W, Yu Q, et al. Molecularly defined and functionally distinct cholinergic subnetworks. Neuron. 2022;**110**(22):3774-3788 e3777. DOI: 10.1016/j.neuron.2022.08.025

[30] Ahmadian SS, Rezvanian A, Peterson M, Weintraub S, Bigio EH, Mesulam MM, et al. Loss of calbindin-D28K is associated with the full range of tangle pathology within basal forebrain cholinergic neurons in Alzheimer's disease. Neurobiology of Aging. 2015;**36**(12):3163-3170. DOI: 10.1016/j.neurobiolaging.2015.09.001

[31] Riascos D, Nicholas A, Samaeekia R, Yukhananov R, Mesulam MM, Bigio EH, et al. Alterations of Ca(2)(+)-responsive proteins within cholinergic neurons in aging and Alzheimer's disease. Neurobiology of Aging. 2014;**35**(6):1325-1333. DOI: 10.1016/j.neurobiolaging.2013.12.017

[32] Price JL, Stern R. Individual cells in the nucleus basalis--diagonal band complex have restricted axonal projections to the cerebral cortex in the rat. Brain Research. 1983;**269**(2):352-356. DOI: 10.1016/0006-8993(83)90145-2

[33] Chaves-Coira I, Martin-Cortecero J, Nunez A, Rodrigo-Angulo ML. Basal forebrain nuclei display distinct projecting pathways and functional circuits to sensory primary and prefrontal cortices in the rat. Frontiers in Neuroanatomy. 2018;**12**:69. DOI: 10.3389/fnana.2018.00069

[34] Robert B, Kimchi EY, Watanabe Y, Chakoma T, Jing M, Li Y, et al. A functional topography within the cholinergic basal forebrain for encoding sensory cues and behavioral reinforcement outcomes. eLife. 2021;**10**. DOI: 10.7554/eLife.69514

[35] Gulledge AT, Bucci DJ, Zhang SS, Matsui M, Yeh HH. M1 receptors mediate cholinergic modulation of excitability in neocortical pyramidal neurons. The Journal of Neuroscience. 2009;**29**(31):9888-9902. DOI: 10.1523/JNEUROSCI.1366-09.2009

[36] Wallace TL, Bertrand D. Importance of the nicotinic acetylcholine receptor system in the prefrontal cortex. Biochemical Pharmacology. 2013;**85**(12):1713-1720. DOI: 10.1016/j.bcp.2013.04.001

[37] Bloem B, Poorthuis RB, Mansvelder HD. Cholinergic modulation of the medial prefrontal cortex: The role of nicotinic receptors in attention and regulation of neuronal activity. Frontiers in Neural Circuits. 2014;**8**:17. DOI: 10.3389/fncir.2014.00017

[38] Hedrick T, Waters J. Acetylcholine excites neocortical pyramidal neurons via nicotinic receptors. Journal of Neurophysiology. 2015;**113**(7):2195-2209. DOI: 10.1152/jn.00716.2014

[39] Poorthuis RB, Bloem B, Schak B, Wester J, de Kock CP, Mansvelder HD. Layer-specific modulation of the prefrontal cortex by nicotinic acetylcholine receptors. Cerebral Cortex. 2013;**23**(1):148-161. DOI: 10.1093/cercor/bhr390

[40] Guillem K, Bloem B, Poorthuis RB, Loos M, Smit AB, Maskos U, et al. Nicotinic acetylcholine receptor beta2 subunits in the medial prefrontal cortex control attention. Science. 2011;**333**(6044):888-891. DOI: 10.1126/science.1207079

[41] Tian MK, Bailey CD, De Biasi M, Picciotto MR, Lambe EK. Plasticity of prefrontal attention circuitry: Upregulated muscarinic excitability in response to decreased nicotinic signaling following deletion of alpha5 or beta2 subunits. The Journal of Neuroscience. 2011;**31**(45):16458-16463. DOI: 10.1523/JNEUROSCI.3600-11.2011

[42] Bailey CD, De Biasi M, Fletcher PJ, Lambe EK. The nicotinic acetylcholine receptor alpha5 subunit plays a key role in attention circuitry and accuracy. The Journal of Neuroscience. 2010;**30**(27):9241-9252. DOI: 10.1523/JNEUROSCI.2258-10.2010

[43] Dani JA. Neuronal nicotinic acetylcholine receptor structure and function and response to nicotine. International Review of Neurobiology. 2015;**124**:3-19. DOI: 10.1016/bs.irn.2015.07.001

[44] Ren JM, Zhang SL, Wang XL, Guan ZZ, Qi XL. Expression levels of the alpha7 nicotinic acetylcholine receptor in the brains of patients with Alzheimer's disease and their effect on synaptic proteins in SH-SY5Y cells. Molecular Medicine Reports. 2020;**22**(3):2063-2075. DOI: 10.3892/mmr.2020.11253

[45] Ma KG, Qian YH. Alpha 7 nicotinic acetylcholine receptor and its effects on Alzheimer's disease. Neuropeptides. 2019;**73**:96-106. DOI: 10.1016/j.npep.2018.12.003

[46] De Jaco A, Bernardini L, Rosati J, Tata AM. Alpha-7 nicotinic receptors in nervous system disorders: From function to therapeutic perspectives. Central Nervous System Agents in Medicinal Chemistry. 2017;**17**(2):100-108. DOI: 10.2174/1871524916666160729111446

[47] Azimi M, Oemisch M, Womelsdorf T. Dissociation of nicotinic alpha7 and alpha4/beta2 sub-receptor agonists for enhancing learning and attentional filtering in nonhuman primates. Psychopharmacology. 2020;**237**(4):997-1010. DOI: 10.1007/s00213-019-05430-w

[48] Hayward A, Adamson L, Neill JC. Partial agonism at the alpha7 nicotinic acetylcholine receptor improves attention, impulsive action and vigilance in low attentive rats. European Neuropsychopharmacology. 2017;**27**(4):325-335. DOI: 10.1016/j.euroneuro.2017.01.013

[49] Bubser M, Byun N, Wood MR, Jones CK. Muscarinic receptor pharmacology and circuitry for the modulation of cognition. Handbook Expression in Pharmacology. 2012;**208**:121-166. DOI: 10.1007/978-3-642-23274-9_7

[50] Yamasaki M, Matsui M, Watanabe M. Preferential localization of muscarinic M1 receptor on dendritic shaft and spine of cortical pyramidal cells and its anatomical evidence for volume transmission. The Journal of Neuroscience. 2010;**30**(12):4408-4418. DOI: 10.1523/JNEUROSCI.5719-09.2010

[51] Caruana DA, Warburton EC, Bashir ZI. Induction of activity-dependent LTD requires muscarinic receptor activation in medial prefrontal cortex. The Journal of Neuroscience. 2011;**31**(50):18464-18478. DOI: 10.1523/JNEUROSCI.4719-11.2011

[52] Romberg C, Bartko S, Wess J, Saksida LM, Bussey TJ. Impaired object-location learning and recognition memory but enhanced sustained attention in M2 muscarinic receptor-deficient mice. Psychopharmacology. 2018;**235**(12):3495-3508. DOI: 10.1007/s00213-018-5065-7

[53] Dillon GM, Shelton D, McKinney AP, Caniga M, Marcus JN,

Ferguson MT, et al. Prefrontal cortex lesions and scopolamine impair attention performance of C57BL/6 mice in a novel 2-choice visual discrimination task. Behavioural Brain Research. 2009;**204**(1):67-76. DOI: 10.1016/j.bbr.2009.04.036

[54] Nicklas PR, Kiefer ML, Whalen MA, Stewart MT, Mosura DE, Bennett EM, et al. Muscarinic M1, but not M4, receptor antagonism impairs divided attention in male rats. Pharmacology, Biochemistry, and Behavior. 2021;**205**:173184. DOI: 10.1016/j.pbb.2021.173184

[55] Kucinski A, Phillips KB, Koshy Cherian A, Sarter M. Rescuing the attentional performance of rats with cholinergic losses by the M1 positive allosteric modulator TAK-071. Psychopharmacology. 2020;**237**(1):137-153. DOI: 10.1007/s00213-019-05354-5

[56] Xie HQ, Leung KW, Chen VP, Chan GK, Xu SL, Guo AJ, et al. PRiMA directs a restricted localization of tetrameric AChE at synapses. Chemico-Biological Interactions. 2010;**187**(1-3):78-83. DOI: 10.1016/j.cbi.2010.02.018

[57] Perrier AL, Massoulie J, Krejci E. PRiMA: The membrane anchor of acetylcholinesterase in the brain. Neuron. 2002;**33**(2):275-285. DOI: 10.1016/s0896-6273(01)00584-0

[58] Dobbertin A, Hrabovska A, Dembele K, Camp S, Taylor P, Krejci E, et al. Targeting of acetylcholinesterase in neurons in vivo: A dual processing function for the proline-rich membrane anchor subunit and the attachment domain on the catalytic subunit. The Journal of Neuroscience. 2009;**29**(14):4519-4530. DOI: 10.1523/JNEUROSCI.3863-08.2009

[59] Xie HQ, Liang D, Leung KW, Chen VP, Zhu KY, Chan WK, et al. Targeting acetylcholinesterase to membrane rafts: A function mediated by the proline-rich membrane anchor (PRiMA) in neurons. The Journal of Biological Chemistry. 2010;**285**(15):11537-11546. DOI: 10.1074/jbc.M109.038711

[60] Perrier NA, Kherif S, Perrier AL, Dumas S, Mallet J, Massoulie J. Expression of PRiMA in the mouse brain: Membrane anchoring and accumulation of 'tailed' acetylcholinesterase. The European Journal of Neuroscience. 2003;**18**(7):1837-1847. DOI: 10.1046/j.1460-9568.2003.02914.x

[61] Balachandran RC, Sieg ML, Tran CTQ, Clancy BM, Beaudin SA, Eubig PA. Cholinergic and dopaminergic interactions alter attention and response inhibition in Long-Evans rats performing the 5-choice serial reaction time task. Pharmacology, Biochemistry, and Behavior. 2018;**175**:160-173. DOI: 10.1016/j.pbb.2018.10.006

[62] Duysen EG, Stribley JA, Fry DL, Hinrichs SH, Lockridge O. Rescue of the acetylcholinesterase knockout mouse by feeding a liquid diet; phenotype of the adult acetylcholinesterase deficient mouse. Brain Research. Developmental Brain Research. 2002;**137**(1):43-54. DOI: 10.1016/s0165-3806(02)00367-x

[63] Farar V, Mohr F, Legrand M, Lamotte d'Incamps B, Cendelin J, Leroy J, et al. Near-complete adaptation of the PRiMA knockout to the lack of central acetylcholinesterase. Journal of Neurochemistry. 2012;**122**(5):1065-1080. DOI: 10.1111/j.1471-4159.2012.07856.x

[64] Vetreno RP, Bohnsack JP, Kusumo H, Liu W, Pandey SC, Crews FT. Neuroimmune and epigenetic involvement in adolescent binge ethanol-induced loss of basal forebrain cholinergic neurons: Restoration with voluntary exercise. Addiction Biology. 2020;**25**(2):e12731. DOI: 10.1111/adb.12731

[65] Hall JM, Gomez-Pinilla F, Savage LM. Nerve growth factor is responsible for exercise-induced recovery of Septohippocampal cholinergic structure and function. Frontiers in Neuroscience. 2018;**12**:773. DOI: 10.3389/fnins.2018.00773

[66] Crews FT, Fisher R, Deason C, Vetreno RP. Loss of basal forebrain cholinergic neurons following adolescent binge ethanol exposure: Recovery with the cholinesterase inhibitor Galantamine. Frontiers in Behavioral Neuroscience. 2021;**15**:652494. DOI: 10.3389/fnbeh.2021.652494

[67] Ke HC, Huang HJ, Liang KC, Hsieh-Li HM. Selective improvement of cognitive function in adult and aged APP/PS1 transgenic mice by continuous non-shock treadmill exercise. Brain Research. 2011;**1403**:1-11. DOI: 10.1016/j.brainres.2011.05.056

[68] Teglas T, Nemeth Z, Koller A, Van der Zee EA, Luiten PGM, Nyakas C. Effects of Long-term moderate intensity exercise on cognitive Behaviors and cholinergic forebrain in the aging rat. Neuroscience. 2019;**411**:65-75. DOI: 10.1016/j.neuroscience.2019.05.037

[69] Xu L, Long J, Su Z, Xu B, Lin M, Chen Y, et al. Restored presynaptic synaptophysin and cholinergic inputs contribute to the protective effects of physical running on spatial memory in aged mice. Neurobiology of Disease. 2019;**132**:104586. DOI: 10.1016/j.nbd.2019.104586

[70] Shamsipour S, Sharifi G, Taghian F. An 8-week Administration of Bifidobacterium bifidum and lactobacillus plantarum combined with exercise training alleviates neurotoxicity of Abeta and spatial learning via acetylcholine in Alzheimer rat model. Journal of Molecular Neuroscience. 2021;**71**(7):1495-1505. DOI: 10.1007/s12031-021-01812-y

[71] Mattson MP, Magnus T. Ageing and neuronal vulnerability. Nature Reviews. Neuroscience. 2006;**7**(4):278-294. DOI: 10.1038/nrn1886

[72] Wu H, Williams J, Nathans J. Complete morphologies of basal forebrain cholinergic neurons in the mouse. eLife. 2014;**3**:e02444. DOI: 10.7554/eLife.02444

[73] Tomasi D, Wiers CE, Manza P, Shokri-Kojori E, Michele-Vera Y, Zhang R, et al. Accelerated aging of the amygdala in alcohol use disorders: Relevance to the dark side of addiction. Cerebral Cortex. 2021;**31**(7):3254-3265. DOI: 10.1093/cercor/bhab006

[74] Woods AJ, Porges EC, Bryant VE, Seider T, Gongvatana A, Kahler CW, et al. Current heavy alcohol consumption is associated with greater cognitive impairment in older adults. Alcoholism, Clinical and Experimental Research. 2016;**40**(11):2435-2444. DOI: 10.1111/acer.13211

[75] Zahr NM, Pohl KM, Saranathan M, Sullivan EV, Pfefferbaum A. Hippocampal subfield CA2+3 exhibits accelerated aging in alcohol use disorder: A preliminary study. Neuroimage Clinic. 2019;**22**:101764. DOI: 10.1016/j.nicl.2019.101764

[76] Rao R, Draper B. Alcohol-related brain damage in older people. Lancet Psychiatry. 2015;**2**(8):674-675. DOI: 10.1016/S2215-0366(15)00215-1

[77] Grant BF, Chou SP, Saha TD, Pickering RP, Kerridge BT, Ruan WJ, et al. Prevalence of 12-month alcohol use, high-risk drinking, and DSM-IV alcohol use disorder in the United States, 2001-2002 to 2012-2013: Results from the National Epidemiologic Survey

on alcohol and related conditions. JAMA Psychiatry. 2017;**74**(9):911-923. DOI: 10.1001/jamapsychiatry.2017.2161

[78] Anttila T, Helkala EL, Viitanen M, Kareholt I, Fratiglioni L, Winblad B, et al. Alcohol drinking in middle age and subsequent risk of mild cognitive impairment and dementia in old age: A prospective population based study. BMJ. 2004;**329**(7465):539. DOI: 10.1136/bmj.38181.418958.BE

[79] Kivipelto M, Rovio S, Ngandu T, Kareholt I, Eskelinen M, Winblad B, et al. Apolipoprotein E epsilon4 magnifies lifestyle risks for dementia: A population-based study. Journal of Cellular and Molecular Medicine. 2008;**12**(6B):2762-2771. DOI: 10.1111/j.1582-4934.2008.00296.x

[80] Barnett A, David E, Rohlman A, Nikolova VD, Moy SS, Vetreno RP, et al. Adolescent binge alcohol enhances early Alzheimer's disease pathology in adulthood through Proinflammatory Neuroimmune activation. Frontiers in Pharmacology. 2022;**13**:884170. DOI: 10.3389/fphar.2022.884170

[81] Hoffman JL, Faccidomo S, Kim M, Taylor SM, Agoglia AE, May AM, et al. Alcohol drinking exacerbates neural and behavioral pathology in the 3xTg-AD mouse model of Alzheimer's disease. International Review of Neurobiology. 2019;**148**:169-230. DOI: 10.1016/bs.irn.2019.10.017

[82] Huang D, Yu M, Yang S, Lou D, Zhou W, Zheng L, et al. Ethanol alters APP processing and aggravates Alzheimer-associated phenotypes. Molecular Neurobiology. 2018;**55**(6):5006-5018. DOI: 10.1007/s12035-017-0703-3

[83] Tucker AE, Alicea Pauneto CDM, Barnett AM, Coleman LG Jr. Chronic ethanol causes persistent increases in Alzheimer's tau pathology in female 3xTg-AD mice: A potential role for lysosomal impairment. Frontiers in Behavioral Neuroscience. 2022;**16**:886634. DOI: 10.3389/fnbeh.2022.886634

[84] Fernandez GM, Lew BJ, Vedder LC, Savage LM. Chronic intermittent ethanol exposure leads to alterations in brain-derived neurotrophic factor within the frontal cortex and impaired behavioral flexibility in both adolescent and adult rats. Neuroscience. 2017;**348**:324-334. DOI: 10.1016/j.neuroscience.2017.02.045

[85] Do Carmo S, Kannel B, Cuello AC. The nerve growth factor metabolic pathway dysregulation as cause of Alzheimer's cholinergic atrophy. Cell. 2021;**11**(1). DOI: 10.3390/cells11010016

[86] Iulita MF, Bistue Millon MB, Pentz R, Aguilar LF, Do Carmo S, Allard S, et al. Differential deregulation of NGF and BDNF neurotrophins in a transgenic rat model of Alzheimer's disease. Neurobiology of Disease. 2017;**108**:307-323. DOI: 10.1016/j.nbd.2017.08.019

[87] Pentz R, Iulita MF, Mikutra-Cencora M, Ducatenzeiler A, Bennett DA, Cuello AC. A new role for matrix metalloproteinase-3 in the NGF metabolic pathway: Proteolysis of mature NGF and sex-specific differences in the continuum of Alzheimer's pathology. Neurobiology of Disease. 2021;**148**:105150. DOI: 10.1016/j.nbd.2020.105150

[88] Perovic M, Tesic V, Mladenovic Djordjevic A, Smiljanic K, Loncarevic-Vasiljkovic N, Ruzdijic S, et al. BDNF transcripts, proBDNF and proNGF, in the cortex and hippocampus throughout the life span of the rat. Age (Dordrecht, Netherlands). 2013;**35**(6):2057-2070. DOI: 10.1007/s11357-012-9495-6

[89] Vecchio I, Sorrentino L, Paoletti A, Marra R, Arbitrio M. The state of the art on acetylcholinesterase inhibitors in the treatment of Alzheimer's disease. Journal of Central Nervous System Diseases. 2021;**13**:11795735211029113. DOI: 10.1177/11795735211029113

[90] Marucci G, Buccioni M, Ben DD, Lambertucci C, Volpini R, Amenta F. Efficacy of acetylcholinesterase inhibitors in Alzheimer's disease. Neuropharmacology. 2021;**190**:108352. DOI: 10.1016/j.neuropharm.2020.108352

[91] Srivastava S, Ahmad R, Khare SK. Alzheimer's disease and its treatment by different approaches: A review. European Journal of Medicinal Chemistry. 2021;**216**:113320. DOI: 10.1016/j.ejmech.2021.113320

[92] Bohnen NI, Kaufer DI, Hendrickson R, Ivanco LS, Lopresti BJ, Koeppe RA, et al. Degree of inhibition of cortical acetylcholinesterase activity and cognitive effects by donepezil treatment in Alzheimer's disease. Journal of Neurology, Neurosurgery, and Psychiatry. 2005;**76**(3):315-319. DOI: 10.1136/jnnp.2004.038729

[93] Moss DE, Perez RG. Anti-neurodegenerative benefits of acetylcholinesterase inhibitors in Alzheimer's disease: Nexus of cholinergic and nerve growth factor dysfunction. Current Alzheimer Research. 2021;**18**(13):1010-1022. DOI: 10.2174/1567205018666211215150547

[94] Petrella JR, Prince SE, Krishnan S, Husn H, Kelley L, Doraiswamy PM. Effects of donepezil on cortical activation in mild cognitive impairment: A pilot double-blind placebo-controlled trial using functional MR imaging. AJNR. American Journal of Neuroradiology. 2009;**30**(2):411-416. DOI: 10.3174/ajnr.A1359

[95] Li W, Antuono PG, Xie C, Chen G, Jones JL, Ward BD, et al. Changes in regional cerebral blood flow and functional connectivity in the cholinergic pathway associated with cognitive performance in subjects with mild Alzheimer's disease after 12-week donepezil treatment. NeuroImage. 2012;**60**(2):1083-1091. DOI: 10.1016/j.neuroimage.2011.12.077

[96] Muller P, Vellage AK, Schmicker M, Menze I, Grothe MJ, Teipel SJ, et al. Structural MRI of the basal forebrain as predictor of cognitive response to galantamine in healthy older adults-a randomized controlled double-blinded crossover study. Alzheimers Dementia (N Y). 2021;**7**(1):e12153. DOI: 10.1002/trc2.12153

[97] Bagaria J, Bagyinszky E, An SSA. Genetics, functions, and clinical impact of Presenilin-1 (PSEN1) gene. International Journal of Molecular Sciences. 2022;**23**(18). DOI: 10.3390/ijms231810970

[98] Bustos V, Pulina MV, Ledo J. Amyloidogenic and anti-amyloidogenic properties of presenilin 1. Advances in Pharmacology. 2021;**90**:239-251. DOI: 10.1016/bs.apha.2020.09.010

[99] Garcia-Ayllon MS, Campanari ML, Montenegro MF, Cuchillo-Ibanez I, Belbin O, Lleo A, et al. Presenilin-1 influences processing of the acetylcholinesterase membrane anchor PRiMA. Neurobiology of Aging. 2014;**35**(7):1526-1536. DOI: 10.1016/j.neurobiolaging.2014.01.147

[100] Jazi R, Lalonde R, Qian S, Strazielle C. Regional brain evaluation of acetylcholinesterase activity in PS1/A246E transgenic mice. Neuroscience Research. 2009;**63**(2):106-114. DOI: 10.1016/j.neures.2008.11.002

[101] Romberg C, Mattson MP, Mughal MR, Bussey TJ, Saksida LM.

Impaired attention in the 3xTgAD mouse model of Alzheimer's disease: Rescue by donepezil (Aricept). The Journal of Neuroscience. 2011;**31**(9):3500-3507. DOI: 10.1523/JNEUROSCI.5242-10.2011

[102] Lindner MD, Hogan JB, Hodges DB Jr, Orie AF, Chen P, Corsa JA, et al. Donepezil primarily attenuates scopolamine-induced deficits in psychomotor function, with moderate effects on simple conditioning and attention, and small effects on working memory and spatial mapping. Psychopharmacology. 2006;**188**(4):629-640. DOI: 10.1007/s00213-006-0556-3

[103] Proulx E, Power SK, Oliver DK, Sargin D, McLaurin J, Lambe EK. Apamin improves prefrontal nicotinic impairment in mouse model of Alzheimer's disease. Cerebral Cortex. 2020;**30**(2):563-574. DOI: 10.1093/cercor/bhz107

[104] Driscoll LL, Carroll JC, Moon J, Crnic LS, Levitsky DA, Strupp BJ. Impaired sustained attention and error-induced stereotypy in the aged Ts65Dn mouse: A mouse model of down syndrome and Alzheimer's disease. Behavioral Neuroscience. 2004;**118**(6):1196-1205. DOI: 10.1037/0735-7044.118.6.1196

[105] Chen GJ, Xiong Z, Yan Z. Abeta impairs nicotinic regulation of inhibitory synaptic transmission and interneuron excitability in prefrontal cortex. Molecular Neurodegeneration. 2013;**8**:3. DOI: 10.1186/1750-1326-8-3

[106] Viel TA, Caetano AL, Albuquerque MS, Araujo MS, Buck HS. Chronic infusion of amyloid-beta peptide and sustained attention altered alpha7 nicotinic receptor density in the rat brain. Current Alzheimer Research. 2012;**9**(10):1210-1220. DOI: 10.2174/156720512804142930

[107] Dwomoh L, Tejeda GS, Tobin AB. Targeting the M1 muscarinic acetylcholine receptor in Alzheimer's disease. Neuronal. Signals. 2022;**6**(1):NS20210004. DOI: 10.1042/NS20210004

[108] Scarr E, McLean C, Dean B. Higher levels of different muscarinic receptors in the cortex and hippocampus from subjects with Alzheimer's disease. Journal of Neural Transmission (Vienna). 2017;**124**(3):273-284. DOI: 10.1007/s00702-016-1625-3

[109] Tsang SW, Lai MK, Kirvell S, Francis PT, Esiri MM, Hope T, et al. Impaired coupling of muscarinic M1 receptors to G-proteins in the neocortex is associated with severity of dementia in Alzheimer's disease. Neurobiology of Aging. 2006;**27**(9):1216-1223. DOI: 10.1016/j.neurobiolaging.2005.07.010

[110] Reitz NL, Nunes PT, Savage LM. Adolescent binge-type ethanol exposure in rats mirrors age-related cognitive decline by suppressing cholinergic tone and hippocampal neurogenesis. Frontiers in Behavioral Neuroscience. 2021;**15**:772857. DOI: 10.3389/fnbeh.2021.772857

[111] Givens B. Effect of ethanol on sustained attention in rats. Psychopharmacology. 1997;**129**(2):135-140. DOI: 10.1007/s002130050173

[112] Spear LP. Consequences of adolescent use of alcohol and other drugs: Studies using rodent models. Neuroscience and Biobehavioral Reviews. 2016;**70**:228-243. DOI: 10.1016/j.neubiorev.2016.07.026

[113] Nunes PT, Kipp BT, Reitz NL, Savage LM. Aging with alcohol-related brain damage: Critical brain circuits associated with cognitive dysfunction. International Review of Neurobiology.

2019;**148**:101-168. DOI: 10.1016/bs.irn.2019.09.002

[114] Sey NYA, Gomez AA, Madayag AC, Boettiger CA, Robinson DL. Adolescent intermittent ethanol impairs behavioral flexibility in a rat foraging task in adulthood. Behavioural Brain Research. 2019;**373**:112085. DOI: 10.1016/j.bbr.2019.112085

[115] Vetreno RP, Broadwater M, Liu W, Spear LP, Crews FT. Adolescent, but not adult, binge ethanol exposure leads to persistent global reductions of choline acetyltransferase expressing neurons in brain. PLoS One. 2014;**9**(11):e113421. DOI: 10.1371/journal.pone.0113421

[116] Sun W, Chen L, Zheng W, Wei X, Wu W, Duysen EG, et al. Study of acetylcholinesterase activity and apoptosis in SH-SY5Y cells and mice exposed to ethanol. Toxicology. 2017;**384**:33-39. DOI: 10.1016/j.tox.2017.04.007

[117] Fernandez GM, Savage LM. Adolescent binge ethanol exposure alters specific forebrain cholinergic cell populations and leads to selective functional deficits in the prefrontal cortex. Neuroscience. 2017;**361**:129-143. DOI: 10.1016/j.neuroscience.2017.08.013

[118] Birrell JM, Brown VJ. Medial frontal cortex mediates perceptual attentional set shifting in the rat. The Journal of Neuroscience. 2000;**20**(11):4320-4324 https://www.ncbi.nlm.nih.gov/pubmed/10818167

[119] Kipp BT, Nunes PT, Savage LM. Sex differences in cholinergic circuits and behavioral disruptions following chronic ethanol exposure with and without thiamine deficiency. Alcoholism, Clinical and Experimental Research. 2021;**45**(5):1013-1027. DOI: 10.1111/acer.14594

[120] Roland JJ, Levinson M, Vetreno RP, Savage LM. Differential effects of systemic and intraseptal administration of the acetylcholinesterase inhibitor tacrine on the recovery of spatial behavior in an animal model of diencephalic amnesia. European Journal of Pharmacology. 2010;**629**(1-3):31-39. DOI: 10.1016/j.ejphar.2009.12.005

Chapter 5

Role of Acetylcholine in Chronic Diseases

Vandana Mohan, Dhirender Kaushik and Komal Arora

Abstract

The complex and extensive network of brain signals plays a vital role in maintaining physiological mechanisms and homeostasis. Acetylcholine, a chief neurotransmitter of the parasympathetic nervous system, is an important component of the cholinergic system along with cholinergic receptors, acetylcholinesterase, and choline acetyltransferase. It is responsible for mediating cell-to-cell communication and regulates various peripheral and non-neuronal cholinergic signals. Any alteration in the levels of acetylcholine leads to chronic diseases. Chronic diseases, the leading causes of disability, require continuing health care, medical attention, and potential therapeutics. This chapter will cover a brief overview of acetylcholine including its synthesis and degradation, the cholinergic system, and the influence of acetylcholine on different chronic diseases including neurological complications, metabolic disorders, cardiac diseases, and immune disorders. Moreover, the mechanistic approach of acetylcholine in different diseases and the therapies for recovering the levels of acetylcholine will be reviewed in this chapter. Further, this will illustrate the acetylcholine interaction with various cells implicated in the diseases. The insights on agonists and antagonists of acetylcholine and different targets of cholinergic receptors that could help to design better strategies to control these chronic diseases will also be provided.

Keywords: acetylcholine, chronic diseases, cholinergic, neurotransmitter, mechanistic approach, parasympathetic nervous system, treatment

1. Introduction

The most common and significant chemical of the nervous system capable of performing numerous roles within the anatomical framework of humans is Acetylcholine (Ach). In particular, it is termed as a chemical messenger liberated via nerve cell for broadcasting signals to other neurons and to other generalized cells, for instance, heart and glandular cells. It is also found at the junctions of neuron and muscles; on the ganglion of visceral motor system and in the numerous spots in Central Nervous System. Acetylcholine, the designated expression has been derived from its structural association as an "ester of acetic acid" and "choline". Cholinergic tissues are those that use or respond to Ach present within a body while the chemicals that interfere with the influence of Ach on the body are referred to as anticholinergics.

Despite the fact of Ach's presence in body's several regions; a myoneural junction has been marked as a normally linked region. At this region, there is a synaptic association between efferent or motor nerve cell and myofiber. Ach is also been able to act as a chemical transmitter between the neurons of pre-ganglion and post-ganglion in an autonomic nervous system [1].

1.1 Biogenesis, retention, and discharge of acetylcholine

1.1.1 Biogenesis

Acetylcholine is produced from choline and acetyl coenzyme A, its two immediate precursors. The choline acetyltransferase (ChAT) enzyme catalyzes the synthesis reaction in a single step.

$$Choline + Acetyl\ coenzyme\ A \leftrightarrow Acetylcholine + Coenzyme\ A \quad (1)$$

ChAT was first detected in 1943 in a cell-free based preparation, and which was cloned and purified from various sources [2]. ChAT purification has enabled the creation of selective antibodies targeted to a particular antigen. The enzyme, acetylcholinesterase (AChE), synthesized by the cells having the site for choline receptors and cholinergic neurons, is in control to degrade acetylcholine. The location of ChAT is mostly present in regions of the brain wherein the production of Ach occurs. ChAT is localized in the nerve endings within cholinergic neurons, but it is also present in axons, in which it is transferred out of its production in the cell body. The sub-cellular fractionation experiments revealed the recovery of ChAT in the synaptosomes and in the synaptosomal complex suggested the cytoplasmic nature of ChAT [3].

Acetyl CoA is generated from pyruvate, which is created from glucose in the mammalian brain. It is unknown how acetyl CoA, which is widely considered to be generated at the inner membrane of the mitochondria, reaches the cytoplasmic ChAT, and this might be a rate-limiting step.

1.1.2 Retention

Following the production of ACh by ChAT at the nerve terminal, ACh is transported to storage receptacles [4]. Vesicular acetylcholine transporter (VAChT) has been cloned and expressed. Because of its sequence, it belongs to the 12-membrane-spanning family of biogenic amine transporters identified in adrenergic nerve terminals [5, 6]. Remarkably, the transporter gene is situated within an intron of the ChAT gene, implying the co-regulation of ChAT and VAChT. A proton-pumping ATPase drives ACh uptake in the vesicle while coupled H+ and ACh counter transport permit the vesicle to maintain iso-osmoticity and electroneutrality [4].

Vesamicol selectively inhibits Ach transport with an IC50 of 40 nM, inhibits vesicular ACh uptake [4–6]. Non-competitive mechanism of inhibition was found for vesamicol which means that it works on a location other than the transporter's ACh-binding site. Further, Vesamicol inhibits the induced release of freshly generated ACh while having no effect on the uptake of choline, synthesis of acetylcholine and high-affinity choline uptake, ACh synthesis, or inflow of calcium ions. The notion that the release of ACh is lost as a result of the vesicle's inhibition of absorption clearly implies that the vesicle is the source of ACh release. Moreover, Vesamicol also inhibits the expressed transporter from the cloned cDNA [5, 6].

1.1.3 Discharge

It is believed that more than 50% of total choline utilized in the production of acetylcholine, is derived straightforwardly from reprocessing of liberated acetylcholine, which is metabolized/hydrolyzed by cholinesterase to choline. This metabolically generated choline is likely to be swiftly absorbed before it diffuses away from the synaptic cleft. The disintegration of phosphatidyl-choline, which may be accelerated due to local production in Ach, is another source of choline. Choline produced from the two mentioned sources turned accessible to the space outside of the cell which is subsequently taken up by the nerve ending with high affinity. Due to the fact that choline is not able to cross blood brain barrier (BBB) when present in plasma, the metabolic origins of choline found to be more significant in the CNS. Accordingly, in the CNS, elevated choline absorption into the neurons of cholinergic system is not maximal or is saturated, suggesting the choline availability as the rate limiting step in the production of acetylcholine.

1.2 Cholinergic system

The cholinergic system consists of organized nerve fibers responsible for projecting nerve impulses, also known as action potentials through acetylcholine. The release of acetylcholine stimulates the nerve impulse during transmission. Memory, selective attention, and emotional processing are among the cognitive activities connected with the cholinergic system.

1.2.1 Cholinergic projections

The widely projecting and local circuits constitute the cholinergic system. The extended projections of cholinergic neurons originate in nuclei of basal forebrain and project throughout the brain. Acetylcholine is transmitted to the cerebral cortex via the "nucleus basalis of Meynert" and the "diagonal band of Broca". There are also cholinergic connections between the nucleus located in septal region and the hippocampus located deep into temporal lobe. The local circuitry of cholinergic system inside corpus striatum (important component of basal ganglia) interacts with neurons of GABA system and nigrostriatal dopamine system engaged in extra-pyramidal movement.

1.2.2 Cholinergic system: the role in cognition

The cholinergic system has been linked to several cognitive functions such as memory, attention, memory, and processing of emotions. Research done on humans and animals indicated that sustained attentional performance has/had been driven by the cholinergic input from the basal forebrain [7]. In general, cholinergic system activation aids better focussed ability to retain the relevant stimuli and filter out the irrevelant ones, but particular projections to the medial prefrontal cortex regulate anxious reactions to contextual cues acetylcholine influences working memory and the attentional processes necessary for error detection by regulating arousal and attention. The cholinergic system is also tightly linked to emotional processing; moreover, the inputs of cholinergic neurons to the frontoparietal cortex modulate the direction of attention toward emotional expression. In view of the fact that the system is governing so many aspects of cognition, diminished cholinergic tone correlated to Alzheimer's disease and leads to poor intellectual execution that includes attentiveness, memory, attention, and executive functioning [8].

1.3 Cholinergic receptors

Nicotinic acetylcholine receptors are ion channels that are activated by a ligand. They are made up of five polypeptide subunits, including 2 α subunits plus β, γ and δ subunits with its further two subtypes viz. Muscular (N1) and Neuronal (N2). N1 consists of α_1, β_1, γ, δ (2:1:1:1) subunits in the case of embryo while α1, β1, δ, and ε (2:1:1:1) in case of adults. N2 possesses 2α, 3β subunits that can form twelve different combinations of nicotinic receptor subunits. When two acetylcholine molecules bind to the nicotinic acetylcholine receptor, there exists a change in the internal conformation of the pentameric structure, forming a trans-membrane aperture that allows the movement of Na^+, K^+ (3 sodium ions out of cells while pumping 2 potassium ions into cells) and Ca^{2+} ions to pass through. Depending on the intensity of the initiating stimulation, the transport of these ions will result in cell depolarization [9].

mAchR, known as "Muscarinic acetylcholine receptors" belong to the subfamily of G-protein coupled receptor (GPCR) complexes, commonly found in brain, bladder, sweat glands, eye and gland, constitute a single polypeptide chain with 7 distinct sections organized in an alpha-helical structure. Hydrophobic residues in these alpha helices permit the polypeptide for spanning the neural membrane about 7 times. The 5th cytoplasmic facing loop along with the carboxy tail of this polypeptide communicates with G-proteins (made of α, β, and γ subunits), also known as secondary messengers. When acetylcholine binds to the muscarinic receptor, there is a change in its configuration, prompting the alpha sub-unit for releasing the naturally attached inactive metabolite (purine nucleotide diphosphate consisting of guanine and pyrophosphate) called guanosine di-phosphate, GDP and swap this for tri-phosphate molecule (guanosine triphosphate, GTP). α subunit dissociates from the distinct components (β and γ) upon binding of triphosphate molecule to alpha component. Further, GTP collaborate in accompany to other signaling proteins. An inherent activity of GTPase in α subunit metabolize GTP again to GDP, thus shutting off the second messenger system over time. Muscarinic receptors have numerous tissue-dependent activities in the physiological system of humans. These activities could be either of two: STIMULATORY or INHIBITORY due to their utilization of secondary messengers to achieve the desired results. M2 and M4, the subtypes of Muscarinic receptor, inhibits adenylate cyclase to function. There is an inhibition of adenylate cyclase by the alpha component of G protein upon binding of Ach to Muscarinic receptor subtypes (M2 or M4) that results in decrement of intra cellular cAMP and as there is an essential role of cAMP in activating/inhibiting the numerous down-stream elements of signaling pathway, it's decreased concentration leads to plethora of pitfalls. The actions of M type subreceptors (M1, M3 & M5) have been carried out via stimulating phospholipase C (PLC). The active complex of G protein communaticate to PLC and activates it that cause hydrolysation of phophatidyl-inositol to Inositol tri-phosphate (IP3) and di-acyl-glycerol (DAG). The increase in intra cellular calcium concentration in the cytoplasm of the cell is due to the interaction of secondary messentar IP3 with its receptors located in SER (Smooth Endoplasmic Reticulum) [10].

2. Influence of acetylcholine on chronic diseases

Acetylcholine, being a mediator of cell to cell communication, and responsible for various peripheral and non-neuronal cholinergic signals. Any alteration in the levels of acetylcholine leads to chronic diseases. The same has been depicted in **Figure 1**.

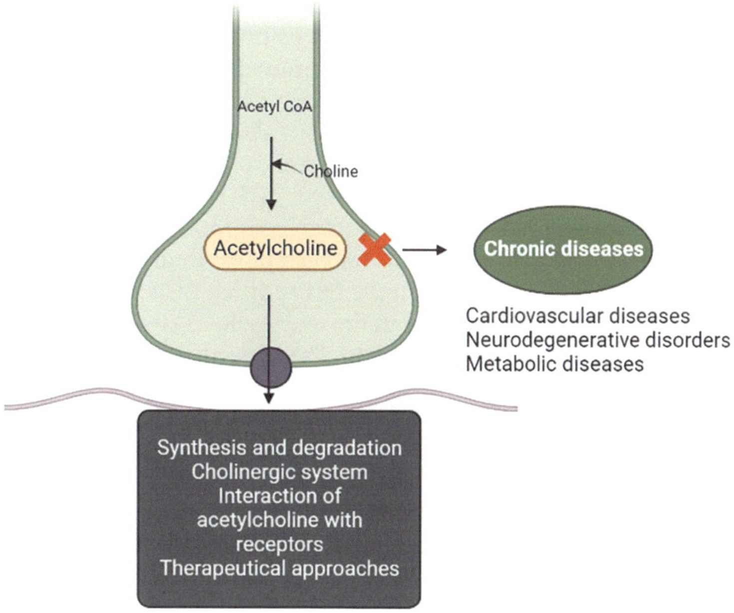

Figure 1.
The graphical illustration of acetylcholine effect on chronic disorders.

2.1 Acetylcholine and cardiovascular system

The heart's purpose is to pump blood to body tissues and organs. Myocardial infarction, being an index event, causes anatomical and physiological changes in the heart, called "cardiac remodeling". These alterations have been seen only at molecular and cellular stages in the cardiomyocyte. Based on the extent of the damage, cardiac remodeling may escalate to heart failure and, eventually, death [11]. Despite significant efforts in understanding the components implicated in how heart failure evolves, the mode of action underlying the phenomenon remains unknown.

ACh is secreted in the heart vie para-sympathetic division of the ANS and frequently serves in offsetting the effects of fight/flight system. A highly innervated heart's atrial valve activates cholinergic system that reduces heart rate, atrioventricular contractility, and node conduction velocities. Although ventricles displayed cholinergic fibers, however their density within ventricles remain substantially lower than in the atrium [12].

ACh has been universally considered as the primary neurotransmitter of parasympathetic nervous system since the Otto Loewi experimental times till present day investigations. The processes involved in its production and release have now been thoroughly elucidated. The operations of choline acetyltransferase (ChAT), which converts acetyl-CoA and choline into ACh in the cytoplasm, are required for ACh synthesis. The vesicular ACh transporter (VAChT) stores cytoplasmic ACh in synaptic vesicles, hence the level of ACh discharged is directly related to the quantity of VAChT. Increased expression of VAChT leads to increased ACh release, whereas decreased VAChT expression leads to decreased ACh release. Ca^{2+} promotes the exocytosis of ACh-filled vesicles by stimulating vesicle fusion with the biological membranes, permitting ACh to be released into the extracellular environment [13].

ACh, being liberated into the extracellular environment, can adhere to nicotinic (nAChR) or muscarinic (mAChR) receptors, activating particular signal transduction series in various types of cells. The muscarinic receptor, a G protein-coupled receptor, is the most important ACh receptor in the heart. The subtypes of Muscarinic receptors (M1–M5) seem to be present all across the systemic circulation and have a range of physiological roles. The most frequent heart's muscarinic receptor subtype is type 2 i.e., AChR-M2). The G-inhibitory (Gi) protein is connected to AChR-M2, whose expression has been thought to counterbalance adrenaline activation via the G-stimulatory (Gs) protein. Cholinesterases, found in the extracellular environment, are present numerously in the heart, break ACh molecules quickly. Incredibly little quantity of ACh persist in the extracellular environment, eliminating the actions of non-receptor-mediated signals. The high-affinity choline transporter transports the choline produced by ACh breakdown again to the cytoplasm of the cell (CHT 1). Considering the fact that ACh-synthesizing cells require choline from the extracellular environment in order to synthesize ACh, CHT1 activity is a step-limiting element in ACh production. The ACh release by heart myocytes reliant on the activity of VAChT. This premise is supported by three pieces of evidence. First, vesicle-like structures were identified to present together in accompany of VAChT in cardiac myocytes. Secondly, knocked out VAChT derived heart myocytes from mice have decreased Ach secretion. Third, ACh was found in the supernatant of in vitro cardiomyocyte preparations, however absent in VAChT mutant animals (cardiac specific) [14].

2.1.1 Cardioprotective actions of Ach

ACh is found to protect the heart against a variety of pathological diseases, including isoproterenol-induced hypertrophy, hypertension, myocardial infarction, chronic chagas cardiomyopathy, and angiotensin II (Ang-II)-induced cardiac dysfunction. Cholinergic signaling was manipulated pharmacologically by using cholinesterase inhibitors such as pyridostigmine (PYR), surgically by modifying vagus nerve activity, or genetically engineered mice models to investigate the influence of variations in cholinergic activity on heart disease development. Cholinergic signaling was modulated pharmacologically with pyridostigmine (PYR), a cholinesterase inhibitor, by modifying the activity of vagus nerve with surgical procedures, or genetically engineered mouse models to examine the effect of alterations in cholinergic activity on the development of heart disease. In infarcted mice, eating improved hemodynamic measures, autonomic balance, and ventricular dysfunction. Likewise, Gavioli and colleagues discovered that PYR therapy decreased heart hypertrophy and ventricular dysfunction in two different animal models of hyperadrenergic stimulation. Even though these research findings consistently demonstrated that PYR therapies provide cardio protection in various mouse injury models, it could be fascinating to determine for certain if PYR's potential benefits have been recognized massively in human patients. In this spirit, the Alzheimer's pateints who intake the inhibitors of cholinesterase are at lower risk of mortality. The study by Li et al. described how chronic heart diseased rats survived upon the stimulation of vagus nerve. Although stimulated nerve had no effect on infarct size, it did enhance the functionality of cardiac cell and decrease hypertrophic cardiomyopathy. It is important to note here that rats whose nerve got stimulated survived 70% more compared to those that were not stimulated. Vaseghi et al. demonstrated in another work employing infarcted pigs that stimulated vagus nerve enhanced the "rest and digest" system and decreased abnormal heart rhythms of the ventricles, most likely by stabilizing the infarct border zones [15].

In conclusion, growing evidence suggests that cardiac cholinergic transmission (both neuronal and non-neuronal) has a biological purpose in damaged conditions, despite the fact that considerations for every ACh generator to recovery remains to be firmly defined yet.

2.2 Acetylcholine and neurodegenerative diseases

2.2.1 Alzheimer's disease

Alzheimer's disease (AD) is a neurodegenerative, inevitable, progressive disorder that affects memory, thinking behavior and other potential activities, the early symptoms of which include trouble in recalling recent talks, names or events; depression; lack of interest (apathy) and later signs are confusion, hindered communication, disorientation, behavioral changes and poor judgment [16]. Because the cholinergic system is disrupted in this condition, the "cholinergic hypothesis" was proposed. Cholinergic innervation may be disrupted even in the early stages of Alzheimer's disease, according to researchers. Neurons of nucleus basalis are especially vulnerable to this degradation. It is widely accepted about the functionality of cholinergic system that could be increased utilizing the Nicotinic/muscarinic receptor agonists and antagonists, thus these two approaches have been into action to treat Alzheimer disease. The hyperactivity of AChE produces a drop in the levels of Ach, leading to cholinergic system degeneration. The usage of acetylcholinesterase inhibitors may enhance a patient's life; however, these medications are merely indicative, meaning it results in the delaying of symptom onset, thus cannot be considered as definitive treatment. AChE activity assessments is of little relevance in the initial phases of the disease since only a small reduction in its effects has been seen. AChE is found in both the main cleft and the postjunctional fold, however the majority of it is found in the basal lamina. The location of AChE is in close proximity to the surface of a muscle as compared to the pre-synaptic layer present in the main cleft, but it is present along the whole stretch of the postjunctional fold, reaching its highest concentration down past the fold. According to research, the alterations in early AD are presynaptic. This is consistent with prior research, which found that AChE activity declines very little in early illness. Neuronal apoptosis occurs over time in Alzheimer's disease. AChE may potentially have a role in this. The tissues having more concentration of AChE are more vulnerable to apoptosis. In one of the study Tau Glycoge synthase kinase 3 (GSK3) was activated by the transfection of N-AChE-S in cell culture. GSK3 caused the tau hyperphosphorylation and apoptotic induction [17]. The amyloid hypothesis is another effort to explain the etiology of AD. Its supporters claim that the illness is caused by the buildup of protein called beta amyloid (AB) in brain. It is also thought about the neurodegeneration and symptom manifestations by these AB deposits. Amyloid beta is neurotoxic to mature neurons, causing them to die. Amyloid beta is generated by proteolysis of amyloid precursor protein (endosomal/lysosomal/at the plasma membrane surface) (APP). This process is triggered by the presence of alpha secretase (unit of preselin 1). AChE has also been found to participate in beta amyloid buildup. AChE has variable sensitivity to inhibitors in Alzheimer's disease, inhibited by indoleamine and bacitracin [18]. Furthermore, this enzyme can directly communicate with beta amyloid. The amyloid beta-AChE complex is more hazardous to the brain than only the aggregates of beta amyloid [19].

2.2.2 Parkinson's disease

Parkinson's disease (PD) is a kind of neurological disorder. After Alzheimer's disease, it is the second most prevalent neurodegenerative disease. This illness is hypothesized to be caused by Lewy body (LB) and neurite aggregates. They accumulate inside "substantia nigra" (SN) & gradually degenerate the system producing dopamine neurons via neuronal destruction. The manifestations arise after half of the neurons deteriorate. Parkinson's disease also results in the malfunctioning of the cholinergic system, causing weakening of Meynert basalis nucleus, other cognitive disfigurements and hence dementia. Cholinergic deficiencies are more evident in Parkinson's disease than in Alzheimer's disease [20]. AChE activity decreases significantly with Parkinson's disease. This decline is due to the degeneration of cholinergic neurons which has decreased independently of any movement action and illness severity. Dementia patients have greater impairment in AChE activity. The individuals who were not reported with dementia but with a lower concentration of AChE in outer layer of the cerebrum have been found to have low intellectual disability, which coincides with the degradation of neurons producing choline. This association, though, varies. The number of cholinergic terminals was reduced in around one-third of the individuals. An association of various brain's areas in Parkinson's disease results in a wide range of apparent symptoms. The vulnerability of degrading choline-producing neurons of neo-cortex is more in men as compared to women [21]. An early buildup of α-synuclein in cholinergic neurons in the basal forebrain has been linked to the development of LB and neuronal loss in the SN. AChE activity was also shown to be decreased in individuals with early Parkinson's disease dementia, namely in the cerebellar medial occipital cortex. This is the location with the most cholinergic denervation. Cholinergic denervation adds to depressed symptoms in Parkinson's disease. It becomes more obvious, however, when the patient also develops dementia. βA deposits are also significant in the pathogenesis of Parkinson's disease. As previously stated, AChE may play an essential role in deposition of βA in the brain. It is probable that it will also improve Amyloid beta aggregation in Parkinson's disease. Postural instability and gait difficulties are motor subtypes in Parkinson's disease (PIGD). This kind of Parkinson's disease is distinguished by a limited sensitivity to dopaminergic medications. PIGD is one of the elements that contribute to the development of dementia. This subtype frequently has an accumulation of βA in the brain, which magnifies cognitive deficits in addition to those attributed with PIGD. It has also been demonstrated that βA deposition in Parkinson's disease patients might independently worsen apathy. In these cases, there was a strong association betweenβ A binding and apathy [22]. βA might be deposited in both the cerebral cortex and the striatum. Gait disruption in Parkinson's disease is linked to cholinergic deficiencies in the basal forebrain and an increased risk of cognitive loss. Gait speed was correlated in patients with cholinergic and dopaminergic degeneration. Furthermore, cortical AChE activity was lower than normal in certain cases. Impaired postural control and gait abnormalities are related with pedunculopontine nucleus dysfunction. Increased postural sway is related with reduced cholinergic innervation of the thalamus and, as a result, lower AChE activity. In Parkinson's disease, p-tau is also deposited. Deposition of this molecule/protein have been found in the olfactory bulb of up to 80% of Parkinson's disease patients. Its buildup is most likely linked to cognitive deterioration and the progression of dementia in patients with idiopathic Parkinson's disease. AChE increases the formation of p-tau in the brain.

Acetylcholinesterase, furthermore, contribute significantly to the development of ocular disorders. The favorable effect has been observed on retinal development after inhibition [23]. Visual abnormalities occur in Parkinson's disease, with reasons spanning from the retina to higher cortical parts of the brain. Dopamine insufficiency is assumed to be the primary cause of the retinal alterations. Furthermore, it is not ruled out that AChE may have a role in the pathophysiology of ocular abnormalities in Parkinson's disease. Several mutations, including those in the LRRK2 and DJ-1 genes, can alter the course and onset of Parkinson's disease. In hereditary Parkinsonism, mutations in the LRRK2 gene are prevalent. It is passed down in an autosomal dominant manner. In clinical practise, this type of Parkinson's disease is not distinguishable from idiopathic Parkinson's disease. LRRK2 is involved in inflammation. The activity of AChE in carriers of this mutation was compared to that of AChE in individuals with idiopathic Parkinson's disease. AChE activity was shown to be considerably greater in LRRK2 gene mutation carriers. This is consistent with patients who carry this mutation having a shorter illness course and hence fewer severe non-motor symptoms. Enhanced AChE activity has been linked to increased neurotransmission at cholinergic synapses in the thalamus and cerebellar cortex. It is true that oxidative stress plays a crucial role in the etiology of Parkinson's disease. Its primary cause is glial cell activation. AChE receptor is the most likely type responsible for oxidative stress. Stress causes an increase in AChE by increasing the expression of this type. The rise in AChE-R is mostly due to astrocytes. In Parkinson's disease, AChE is implicated in neuronal death via apoptosis [24]. AChE expression increased in PC12 model cells for Parkinson's disease and SNpc in a mouse model. A lack of the enzyme reduced dopaminergic neuron death.

2.2.3 Huntington's disease

Huntington's disease (HD) is another neurological disorder. It is passed down to progeny as "autosomal dominant" manner. The trigger in IT15 gene (found on the short arm of chromosome 4) results in HD. Mutated IT15 gene encodes "Huntingtin" (HTT) protein that builds up inside tissues, causing the deterioration of nerve cell, which eventually leads to death. The mutation increases the amount of "CAG repeats", that causes the prolonged chain of glutamine (Q) giving polychain Q of greater than 36 toward its anionic terminal. The number of repetitions is inversely proportionate to the age at which the sickness manifests itself. After around 15–20 years, the condition causes cachexia and death. Chorea-like motions, cognitive impairment, and mood disturbances are among the symptoms [25]. It has been discovered that in HD, there is a decline in the production of genes and proteins in this system, rather than a loss of cholinergic neurons. It was demonstrated that AChE activity was lowered in mouse models of HD (R6/1), and as a result, they showed cognitive abnormalities in the middle stage of the illness. Activation of microglial cells has been observed in the carriers of mutation that can be diagnosed 15 years prior to the beginning of HD. Furthermore, activation of these cells coincides with striatal neuron dysfunction. By secreting proinflammatory cytokines, microglia may activate A1 astrocytes [26]. Furthermore, it has been demonstrated that thalamostriatal degeneration may lead to dystonia in HD. It has also been proposed that the cholinergic system is implicated in dystonia. Cholinergic transmission has been established repeatedly in HD. However, it has been proposed that therapy with AChE inhibitors is not recommended in HD [27].

2.2.4 Multiple sclerosis

Multiple sclerosis is an usual de-myelinating disorder of the central nervous system (CNS). Multiple, diffuse autoimmune inflammatory alterations contribute to myelin and oligodendrocyte destruction in SM. T-lymphocytes (mostly CD8+) dominate the inflammatory cell infiltrates. Neurotransmission has been disrupted. Axons are preserved at an initial phases of illness, but they have been irreparably destroyed with increasing time. Inflammatory alterations are dynamic and occur mostly in the substantia alba, also called as white matter. Remyelination occurs at all phases of SM, although mostly during the quiescent period [28]. SM causes a rise in proinflammatory cytokines. AChE activity was shown to be higher for those that possessed this condition compared to the reference healthy population. The effect of AChE has been linked to low levels of ACh and persistent inflammatory diseases. According to investigations, periphery acetyl-cholinesterase action has been a supplementary metric for assessing the "non-neuronal cholinergic system's" functionality in inflammation regulation. The patients suffering from relapsing-remitting SM type (RR-SM), lower ACh levels were associated with higher levels of pro-inflammatory cytokines such as IL-17 and IL1 in both CSF and blood. There is an inverse relation reported between the Ach and AChE in RR-SM patients. More the activity of AChE, less the level of Ach. Furthermore, AChE transcript expression increased. When the individuals with RR-SM were differentiated by the reference group, the enzyme level rose by more than 60%. The enhanced serum AChE activity was caused by its G4 form. Every element that is required for the production of Acetylcholine was unchanged in SM patients, demonstrating that cholinesterases are to blame in generating low levels of Ach. Moreover, greater effect of AChE was linked to elevated concentrations of variety of interleukins (IL-12, 18 and 23) and Tumor necrosis factor. The inflammation of myelin sheath promotes cholinergic dysfunction, which contributes to SM. Because ACh levels alter cytokine levels, uncontrolled metabolism of acetylcholine could be an another pathogenic cause of SM [29]. An imbalance of cholinergic activity has also been detected in the hippocampus of SM patients. This is consistent with some persons experiencing a range of cognitive deficits as a result of this medical issue. In the hippocampus of the patients investigated, ACh levels were lower, ChAT activity was lower, but AChE activity remained same. These diseases may be caused by hyper action of AChE in proportion to the chemical messenger (Ach). Another research found that AChE activity remained constant upon comparing to the reference population. Individuals suffering from SM, on the other hand, showed considerable intellectual disability already. The hike in glial AChE levels has been hypothesized for the cognitive decline that compensated for neuronal AChE's drop. That might explicate the negative association between AChE activity and the neuropsychological examination results, that could suggest a increased response of glial cells in individuals with larger cognitive impairments, according to these researchers. Furthermore, cholinergic equilibrium within AChE & ChAT has been well recognized during the remission period [30]. There is a rise in ChAT and a reduction in AChE at this stage of SM. This balance is reversed in the acute phase of the illness, with AChE hike and reduced ChAT.

2.2.5 Amyotrophic lateral sclerosis

Amyotrophic lateral sclerosis (ALS) is a neurological disorder. The degeneration of nerves occurs in the brain stem, pathways of the cortico-spinal route, and in the horn cells of the anterior region, which results in manifestations that are either motor or non-motor. However, the illness' etiology is still unclear. ALS is more prominent in individuals of ages between 50 and 75 years. The risk of ALS reduces beyond the age of 75 years. Neuronal loss was accompanied by the responses of inflammation entailing the growth of microglial and astrocytic cells in both ALS patients and animals. The defining hallmark of ALS is accumulation of the malfunctioning protein, TDP-43. This protein is generally found in the nucleus of the cell. TDP-43 abnormal folding results in the deposition of aggregates in the cytoplasm, resulting in the motor deficits and disrupted transcriptional process. The condition begins locally and later spreads [31, 32]. This enzyme was created as a consequence of overactive motor neurons. An inflammatory response is prevalent as ALS progresses which leads to an increase in pro-inflammatory cytokines including Interleukins (IL-1, 6), Tumor necrosis factor-alpha, and Interferon alpha [33]. Further, in ALS, there is a presence of microglial cells and reactive astrocytes. Excessive oxidative stress is also present in ALS [34]. R-AChE plays an important function in oxidative stress; however, its source might be reactive astrocytes. This molecular type of AChE may have a role in the development and pathophysiology of ALS.

2.3 Acetylcholine and metabolic diseases

2.3.1 Diabetes

Type 1 diabetes (T1D) is an autoimmune condition characterized by autoreactive T lymphocytes destroying insulin-producing -cells in the pancreatic islets of Langerhans. The illness begins with the loss of -cells in individuals with a genetic predisposition and under particular environmental conditions, followed by the migration and activation of inflammatory cells (T and B cells, myeloid, and natural killer cells) to the islets, resulting in insulitis [35]. The vagus nerve innervates the pancreas via parasympathetic nerve terminals that produce the neurotransmitter acetylcholine (ACh). ACh, in turn, can bind to the nAChRs and mAChRs expressed on pancreatic cells, controlling pancreatic metabolic activities such as glucose homeostasis. Increased vagal activity stimulates insulin production by activating mAChRs on pancreatic cells. Although -cells appear to express a variety of muscarinic receptor subtypes, M3 mAChR is the most numerous and the one that mediates insulin release. M3 mAChR of pancreatic cells deficient mice had poor glucose tolerance and considerably lower insulin secretion. Mice overexpressing pancreatic M3 mAChR, on the other hand, had increased glucose tolerance and insulin production. There is additional evidence that pancreatic -cells functionally express distinct nAChR subunits although the role of these receptors in -cell function is still debated. While some studies found that nAChR agonists had no effect on hyperglycemia or -cell function, others found that administering particular 7nAChR agonists lowered hyperglycemia in diabetic animal models [36]. The vagus nerve also connects the central nervous system and the immune system via the cholinergic anti-inflammatory pathway, where ACh inhibits the production of pro-inflammatory cytokines (TNF, IL-6, HMGB1), reducing the inflammatory response in sepsis and inflammatory disorders. The 7nAChR, in particular, has been linked to the suppression of pro-inflammatory cytokine production by macrophages, as well as other immunological processes such as T cell death and the suppressive activity of T regulatory cells. In addition, the presence of a cholinergic system in non-neuronal cells, including immunocompetent cells, has been well established. These cells include the enzymes choline acetyltransferase

(Chat) and acetylcholinesterase (AChE), as well as the choline transporters required for ACh synthesis. Furthermore, immune cells express both muscarinic and nicotinic ACh receptors, suggesting that the cholinergic system is involved in immune response control. The 7nAChR is expressed on neutrophils, macrophages, B and T cells, and dendritic cells, as well as enterocytes, endothelium, and microglial cells, and has been linked to the pathophysiology of autoimmune disorders. Activating the cholinergic nerve system with particular acetylcholinesterase inhibitors (AChEI) prevents the occurence of hyperglycemia and experimental diabetes [36].

2.3.2 Diabetes heart disease

Diabetes heart disease (DHD) is the leading cause of mortality in diabetics, accounting for more than 80% of fatalities. This high fatality rate is notable in light of major advances in modern health-care systems and diabetes therapy. Insulin sensitivity and metabolic disturbances in type 2 diabetes mellitus (T2DM) restrict glucose homeostasis in the heart by downregulating the expression of glucose transporter-4 (GLUT-4). Continued exposure to metabolic changes worsens vascular permeability, leading to coronary artery disease (CAD) and coronary microvascular disease (CMVD). CAD and CMVD reduce coronary artery blood circulation and myocardium perfusion, increasing heart muscle stress and promoting the onset of DHD [37]. Prior literature has shown that cardiomyocytes have a robust inherent cholinergic machinery called the non-neuronal cholinergic system (NNCS). The NNCS in cardiomyocytes is made up of many components that work together to keep acetylcholine (ACh) homeostasis and allow ACh to serve as an autocrine/paracrine mediator. These components are choline acetyltransferase (ChAT) to synthesize ACh; choline transporter1 (CHT1) for the reuptake of choline into the cardiomyocytes for ACh synthesis; vesicular ACh transporter (VAChT) to store and release ACh; acetylcholinesterase (AChE) to degrade ACh in the extracellular space as well as type-2 muscarinic ACh receptor (M2AChR) for ACh binding and signal transduction. ACh secreted by cardiomyocytes functions as an autocrine/paracrine mediator. Its interaction with M2AChR activates the pro-survival phosphatidylinositol-3-kinase (PI3K)/protein kinase B (Akt)/hypoxia-inducible factor 1-alpha (HIF1) signaling cascade. It has been observed that activating this pathway increases the activation of downstream effectors such as (1) glucose transporter-4 (GLUT-4) to promote glucose absorption and energy preservation and (2) vascular endothelial growth factor (VEGF) to promote angiogenesis. However, the role of cardiac NNCS in DHD pathogenesis is uncertain. This is especially important since diabetes is linked to impaired glucose homeostasis, cell survival, and angiogenesis [38].

2.3.3 Adipose tissue dysfunction (obesity-related diseases)

The nicotinic acetylcholine receptor 3 subtype (3-nAChR) is essential for controlling inflammatory responses. Inflammation causes adipose tissue malfunction, which raises a likelihood of cardiac and metabolic illness.

Obesity is now recognized as a key contributor to a variety of chronic illnesses, incorporating inflammatory & blood-vascular & disorders [39]. Increase in the body's most efficient energy storage tissue called White Adipose Tissue (WAT) leads to obesity because of the fact that WAT produces adipokines. These adipokines are responsible for several pathological processes like inflammation and insulin resistance. Furthermore, obesity causes aberrant productions of inflammatory cytokines and other adipokines from WAT, which can be interpreted as adipose tissue malfunction. Obesity-induced adipose tissue dysfunction always results in persistent low-grade inflammation, which frequently leads to poor organ connections and metabolic abnormalities in various tissues. Indeed, adipose tissue inflammation has been linked to cardiovascular disease and insulin resistance. Diverse adipokines generated by adipose tissue can also alter liver, skeletal muscle, and cardiac functions. Nicotinic acetylcholine receptors (nAChRs) are integral membrane proteins that are members of the ligand-gated ion channel superfamily that mediates and/or modulates cellular signaling. nAChRs are generated in mammals by the assembly of particular combinations of five transmembrane subunits chosen from a pool of 16 homologous polypeptides (α1-7, α9-10, β1-4, δ, ε, γ). Various physiological activities may be mediated by nAChRs assembled with different subunits. It has been proposed that nAChRs, particularly 7-nAChR, play a key regulatory role in the cholinergic anti-inflammatory pathway. The role of nAChRs in regulating adipose tissue functions has also been investigated. TNF- alpha (tumor necrosis factor) production from adipocytes was lowered by activating nAChRs, indicating that nAChRs may alleviate adipose inflammation. Bai et al. hypothesized that in high-fat diet-fed ApoE/mice with 3-nAChR blocked and in IL-6-stimulated adipocytes with α3-nAChR gene silenced, the productions of leptin, resistin, triglyceride, cholesterol, and low-density lipoprotein were significantly increased, but the generations of adiponectin and high-density lipoprotein were significantly deceased [40]. Meanwhile, inflammatory cytokine production was significantly increased. Furthermore, JAK2/STAT3 activation was engaged in the α3-nAChR-dependent signaling pathways in the control of adipose tissue dysfunction.

3. Therapeutics

3.1 Cholinergic agonists and antagonists

Cholinergic agonists including parasympathomimetics, especially muscarinic agonists and cholinergic antagonists encompassing parasympatholytics or muscarinic antagonists are the two categories of medications influencing the parasympathetic nervous system.

3.2 Acetylcholinesterase inhibitors

They are also referred to as anti-cholinesterases that prevent the cholinesterase to disintegrate Ach, hence boosting the amount and intensity of synaptic activity. AChE inhibitors are classified into two types based on their method of action: irreversible and reversible (**Figure 2**). Reversible inhibitors, whether competitive or noncompetitive, have largely medical benefits, whereas irreversible AChE activity modulators have harmful consequences. Reversible AChE inhibitors are crucial in the pharmacological modulation of enzyme activity. These inhibitors include compounds with various functional groups (carbamate, quaternary, or tertiary ammonium group) and have been used in the diagnosis and/or treatment of diseases such as myasthenia gravis, Alzheimer's disease, post-operative ileus, bladder distention, glaucoma, and as an antidote to anticholinergic overdose. Irreversible anticholinesterases comprise organo-phosphates which produce a phosphorylated enzyme that does not regenerate appreciably when hydrolyzed. They have little therapeutic efficacy but are extremely toxicologically significant. Isoflurophate, the most known and investigated chemical

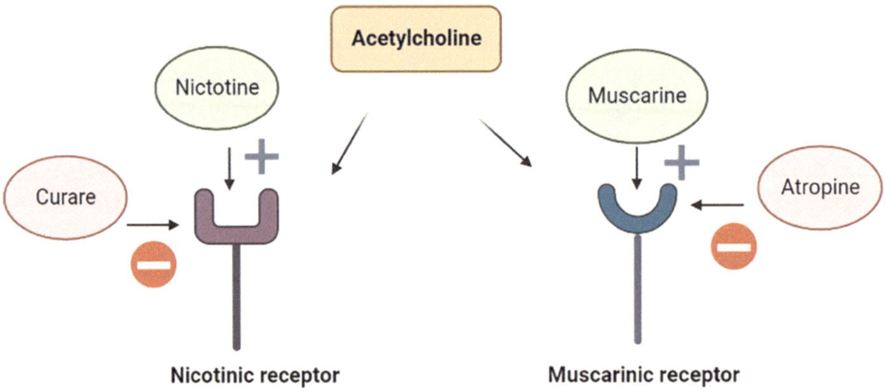

Figure 2.
Agonists and antagonists of acetylcholine.

Inhibitor	Bioactive component/chemical structure	Mechanism of inhibition (reversible/irreversible)
Rivastigmine	Carbamate	Reversible action
Galantamine	Alkaloid	Reversible action
Huperzine A	Alkaloid	Reversible action
7-methoxytacrine	Pyridine derivative	Reversible action
Tacrine	Pyridine derivative	Reversible action
Physostigmine	Carbamate	Reversible action
Pyridostigmine	Carbamate	Reversible action
Aldicarb	Carbamate	Reversible action
Butylate	Carbamate	Reversible action
Diisopropyl Fluorophosphate	Organophosphorous compound	Irreversible action
Trichlorfon	Organophosphorous compound	Irreversible action
Tabun	Organophosphorous compound	Irreversible action
Echothiophate	Organophosphorous compound	Irreversible action
Diazinon	Organophosphorous compound	Irreversible action

Table 1.
Commonly used reversible and irreversible AChE inhibitors.

in this family; malathion, an extensively employed insecticide; echothiophate, among the first substances in this family possesing a therapeutical efficacy; and tabun, the deadly and poisonous nerve gases, are four examples. Some of the commonly used reversible and irreversible inhibitors of Acetylcholinesterase are listed in **Table 1**.

4. Conclusion

Acetylcholine, being a part of cholinergic system, is a neurochemical and capable of performing plethora of functions in brain and human body. In addition to manage the sympathetic, para-sympathetic and autonomic functions, its role in chronic diseases has been well understood and reviewed comprehensively. Furthermore, the cholinergic system, it's projections and the cognitive role has been discussed along with a brief overview of cholinergic receptors. Also, the influence of acetylcholine on different types of chronic diseases including cardiovascular diseases, neurodegenerative disorders and metabolic diseases has been illustrated in detail. In last, the therapeutic section has been presented, covering the insights on agonist and antagonists of Acetylcholine for understanding better treatment options.

Conflict of interest

The authors declare no conflict of interest.

Author details

Vandana Mohan*, Dhirender Kaushik and Komal Arora
Gurugram University, Gurugram, Haryana, India

*Address all correspondence to: vandnakhah@gmail.com

References

[1] Waxenbaum JA, Reddy V, Varacallo M. Anatomy, autonomic nervous system. In: StatPearls [Internet]. Treasure Island (FL): StatPearls Publishing; 2021

[2] Wu D, Hersh LB. Choline acetyltransferase: Celebrating its fiftieth year. Journal of Neurochemistry. 1994; **62**:1653-1663

[3] Taylor P, Brown JH. In: Brady S, Siegel G, Albers RW, Price DL, editors. Basic Neurochemistry: Molecular, Cellular and Medical Aspects. United States: Elsevier; 2005

[4] Parsons SM, Bahr BA, Gracz M, et al. Acetylcholine transport: Fundamental properties and effects of pharmacologic agents. Annals of the New York Academy of Sciences. 1987;**493**:220-233

[5] Erickson JD, Weihe E, Schafer MKM, et al. The VAChT/ChAT "cholinergic gene locus": New aspects of genetic and vesicular regulation of cholinergic function. Progress in Brain Research. 1996;**109**:69-82

[6] Varoqui H, Mennier F-M, Mennier FA, et al. Expression of the vesicular acetylcholine transporter in mammalian cells. Progress in Brain Research. 1996;**109**:83-95

[7] Sarter M, Givens B, Bruno JP. The cognitive neuroscience of sustained attention: Where top-down meets bottom-up. Brain Research. Brain Research Reviews. 2001;**35**(2):146-160. DOI: 10.1016/s0165-0173(01)00044-3

[8] Bentley P, Vuilleumier P, Thiel C, Driver J, Dolan R. Cholinergic enhancement modulates neural correlates of selective attention and emotional processing. NeuroImage. 2003;**20**:58-70

[9] Zoli M, Pucci S, Vilella A, Gotti C. Neuronal and extraneuronal nicotinic acetylcholine receptors. Current Neuropharmacology. 2018;**16**(4): 338-349

[10] Haga T. Molecular properties of muscarinic acetylcholine receptors. Proceedings of the Japan Academy. Series B, Physical and Biological Sciences. 2013;**89**(6):226-256

[11] Burchfield JS, Xie M, Hill JA. Pathological ventricular remodeling: Mechanisms: Part 1 of 2. Circulation. 2013;**128**:388-400. DOI: 10.1161/ CIRCULATIONAHA.113.001878

[12] Sourkes TL. Acetylcholine—From Vagusstoff to cerebral neurotransmitter. Journal of the History of the Neurosciences. 2009;**18**:47-58. DOI: 10.1080/09647040701632305

[13] Van der Kloot W, Molgó J. Quantal acetylcholine release at the vertebrate neuromuscular junction. Physiological Reviews. 1994;**74**:899-991. DOI: 10.1152/ physrev.1994.74.4.899

[14] Roy A, Fields WC, Rocha-Resende C, Resende RR, Guatimosim S, Prado VF, et al. Cardiomyocyte-secreted acetylcholine is required for maintenance of homeostasis in the heart. The FASEB Journal. 2013;**27**:5072-5082. DOI: 10.1096/fj.13-238279

[15] Rocha-Resende C, da Silva AM, Prado MA, Guatimosim S. Protective and anti-inflammatory effects of acetylcholine in the heart. American Journal of Physiology-Cell Physiology. 2021;**320**(2):C155-C161

[16] Bondi MW, Edmonds EC, Salmon DP. Alzheimer's disease: Past,

present, and future. Journal of the International Neuropsychological Society. 2017;**23**(9–10):818-831. DOI: 10.1017/S135561771700100X

[17] Zhang XJ, Greenberg DS. Acetylcholinesterase involvement in apoptosis. Frontiers in Molecular Neuroscience. 2012;**5**:40. DOI: 10.3389/fnmol.2012.00040

[18] Ciro A, Park J, Burkhard G, Yan N, Geula C. Biochemical differentiation of cholinesterases from normal and Alzheimers disease cortex. Current Alzheimer Research. 2012;**9**:138-143. DOI: 10.2174/156720512799015127

[19] Jean L, Brimijoin S, Vaux DJ. In vivo localization of human acetylcholinesterase-derived species in a β-sheet conformation at the core of senile plaques in Alzheimer's disease. The Journal of Biological Chemistry. 2019;**294**:6253-6272. DOI: 10.1074/jbc.RA118.006230

[20] Guo P, Wang RD, Lian TH, Ding DY, Zhang YN, Zhang WJ, et al. Olfactory dysfunction and its association with neuropathologic proteins in cerebrospinal fluid from patients with Parkinson disease. Frontiers in Aging Neuroscience. 2020;**12**:594324. DOI: 10.3389/fnagi.2020.594324

[21] Bohnen NI, Roytman S, Kanel P, Müller ML, Scott PJ, Frey KA, et al. Progression of regional cortical cholinergic denervation in Parkinson's disease. Brain Communications. 2022;**4**(6):fcac320

[22] Zhou Z, Müller MLTM, Kanel P, Chua J, Kotagal V, Kaufer DI, et al. Apathy rating scores and β-amyloidopathy in patients with Parkinson disease at risk for cognitive decline. Neurology. 2020;**94**:e376-e383. DOI: 10.1212/WNL.0000000000008683

[23] Yi YM, Cai L, Shao Y, Xu M, Yi JL. The protective role of tacrine and donepezil in the retina of acetylcholinesterase knockout mice. International Journal of Ophthalmology. 2015;**8**:884-890. DOI: 10.3980/j.issn.2222-3959.2015.05.06

[24] Zhang X, Lu L, Liu S, Ye W, Wu J, Zhang X. Acetylcholinesterase deficiency decreases apoptosis in dopaminergic neurons in the neurotoxin model of Parkinson's disease. The International Journal of Biochemistry & Cell Biology. 2013;**45**:265-272. DOI: 10.1016/j.biocel.2012.11.015

[25] Ahmad Aziz N, Van Der Burg JMM, Tabrizi SJ, Bernhard LG. Overlap between age-at-onset and disease-progression determinants in Huntington disease. Neurology. 2018;**90**:1127. DOI: 10.1212/WNL.0000000000005690

[26] Liddelow SA, Guttenplan KA, Clarke LE, Bennett FC, Bohlen CJ, Schirmer L, et al. Neurotoxic reactive astrocytes are induced by activated microglia. Nature. 2017;**541**:481-487. DOI: 10.1038/nature21029

[27] Giralt A, Saavedra A, Alberch J, Pérez-Navarro E. Cognitive dysfunction in Huntington's disease: Humans, mouse models and molecular mechanisms. Journal of Huntington's Disease. 2012;**1**:155-173. DOI: 10.3233/JHD-120023

[28] Dobson R, Giovannoni G. Multiple sclerosis—A review. European Journal of Neurology. 2019;**26**:27-40. DOI: 10.1111/ene.13819

[29] Gatta V, Mengod G, Reale M, Tata AM. Possible correlation between cholinergic system alterations and

neuro/inflammation in multiple sclerosis. Biomedicine. 2020;**8**:153. DOI: 10.3390/biomedicines8060153

[30] Di Pinto G, Di Bari M, Martin-Alvarez R, Sperduti S, Serrano-Acedo S, Gatta V, et al. Comparative study of the expression of cholinergic system components in the CNS of experimental autoimmune encephalomyelitis mice: Acute vs remitting phase. The European Journal of Neuroscience. 2018;**48**: 2165-2181. DOI: 10.1111/ejn.14125

[31] van Es MA, Hardiman O, Chio A, Al-Chalabi A, Pasterkamp RJ, Veldink JH, et al. Amyotrophic lateral sclerosis. Lancet. 2017;**390**:2084-2098. DOI: 10.1016/S0140-6736(17)31287-4

[32] Hardiman O, Al-Chalabi A, Chio A, Corr EM, Logroscino G, Robberecht W, et al. Amyotrophic lateral sclerosis. Nature Reviews. Disease Primers. 2017;**3**: 1-19. DOI: 10.1038/nrdp.2017.71

[33] Chen X, Hu Y, Cao Z, Liu Q, Cheng Y. Cerebrospinal fluid inflammatory cytokine aberrations in Alzheimer's disease, Parkinson's disease and amyotrophic lateral sclerosis: A systematic review and meta-analysis. Frontiers in Immunology. 2018;**9**:2122. DOI: 10.3389/fimmu.2018.02122

[34] Gerber YN, Sabourin JC, Rabano M, Vivanco MDM, Perrin FE. Early functional deficit and microglial disturbances in a mouse model of amyotrophic lateral sclerosis. PLoS One. 2012;**7**:e36000. DOI: 10.1371/journal.pone.0036000

[35] Meglio AD, Molina BE, Oram RA. Type 1 diabetes. Lancet. The Lancet. 2018;**391**(10138):2449-2462

[36] Fernández-Cabezudo MJ, George JA, Bashir G, Mohamed YA, Al-Mansori A, Qureshi MM, et al. Involvement of acetylcholine receptors in cholinergic pathway-mediated protection against autoimmune diabetes. Frontiers in Immunology. 2019;**10**:1038

[37] Iismaa TP, Kerr EA, Wilson JR, Carpenter L, Sims N, Biden TJ. Quantitative and functional characterization of muscarinic receptor subtypes in insulin-secreting cell lines and rat pancreatic islets. Diabetes. 2000; **49**:392-398. DOI: 10.2337/diabetes.49.3.392

[38] Saw EL, Pearson JT, Schwenke DO, Munasinghe PE, Tsuchimochi H, Rawal S, et al. Activation of the cardiac non-neuronal cholinergic system prevents the development of diabetes-associated cardiovascular complications. Cardiovascular Diabetology. 2021;**20**(1): 1-6

[39] Egom EE. LDL-cholesterol and atherosclerotic cardiovascular disease: Innocent bystander or essential ingredient. Journal of the American College of Cardiology. 2018;**71**(6): 705-706

[40] Bai X, Ju H, Gao L, Xiong Y, Dai R, Huang X, et al. Regulation of nicotinic acetylcholine receptor α3 subtype in adipose tissue dysfunction. Prostaglandins & Other Lipid Mediators. 2019;**142**:53-58. DOI: 10.1016/j.prostaglandins.2019.04.001

Section 2

Acetylcholine Esterase, Neurotoxin

Chapter 6

Paraoxonase in Nervous System

Mohit Vijay Rojekar, Kaushalraj Sunil Dandegonker and Swati Ghanghurde

Abstract

The paraoxonase (PON) family consists of—PON1, PON2 and PON3 which are anti-oxidative, any dysfunction in their action, has been suggested to play a role in the pathobiology of diseases having a chronic inflammatory component. PON1 is the most studied which has paraoxonase, arylesterase, thiolactonase, and anti-oxidant actions. Studies have shown the association between lowered PON1 activity and increased incidence of ischemic stroke, dementia, Parkinson disease, multiple sclerosis, and amyotrophic lateral sclerosis. It may occur due to increased oxidative stress and/or prolonged exposure to organophosphates, and reduced capacity of the body to counter these stresses due to reduced PON1 function. PON2 has arylesterase, lactonase, and antioxidant properties. Under-expression of PON2 is associated with Parkinson Disease and Amyotrophic Lateral Sclerosis, and over-expression with tumors with glioblastoma. Various mechanisms have been proposed for the role of PON2 in the pathobiology of the said diseases. PON3 is least studied. The PON family, to some extent, interacts with acetylcholine esterase (AChE), as both share the same locus, and PONs degrade the inhibitors of AChE, especially the organophosphates. This could probably have significant role in the development of Parkinson disease and the prognosis of the treatment of Alzheimer disease by AChE inhibitors.

Keywords: paraoxonase, arylesterase, lactonase, nervous system, PON1, PON2, PON3

1. Introduction

The paraoxonase (PON) multi-gene family consists of three enzymes: PON1, PON2 and PON3, the genes for which are located adjacent to each other on human chromosome 7q21.22 [1]. The amino acid sequences of the three forms are considerably similar—within the range of 79–95%. All PON genes have nine exons, eight introns and TATA-less promoters. This enzyme came into focus with the notion that PON1 protects low-density lipoproteins (LDL) and high-density lipoproteins (HDL) from lipid peroxidation by the virtue of its arylesterase, lactonase and paraoxonase activities [2]. Paroxonases are HDL-associated, and their antioxidant property plays a vital role in prevention of various microvascular complications due to oxidative stress and also provides protection from various toxic chemicals. All PON family enzymes require calcium to exhibit the action and are able to delay lipid peroxidation in lipoproteins and cell membranes. Thus, polymorphism or any other imbalance in the activity of PON has been suggested to play a role in the pathogenesis of rheumatic diseases, cancers and cardiovascular diseases—i.e. the diseases having a chronic inflammatory component [3, 4]. Although these enzymes have been named paroxonases, the paroxonase activity is significant only for PON1; in others the activity has not been detected. PON1 is a hydrolase and can hydrolyse a wide range of substrates including organophosphorus triester pesticides, lactones, thiolactones, cyclic carbamates, nerve gases like sarin, soman, arylesters, aromatic carboxylic acid and unsaturated aliphatic esters, estrogen-esters, and glucuronide drugs [5].

PON enzymes synthesized in the liver and distributed throughout the human body. They are present in different tissues, and are associated with cell membranes and some lipoproteins, although literature reports free enzyme found in the blood. Paroxonases were named after the ability of PON1 (first to be discovered) to hydrolyze paraoxon, a compound of the organophosphate insecticides class, to the metabolite p-nitrophenol. In vivo, paraoxon, the most toxic form, is an oxidized product of biotransformation of parathion, organophosphate insecticide in the context of which it was found first. As explained above, the name can be said to be a misnomer.

Of the three members of the family, PON1 is the most studied one. It is a circulating Ca^{2+} dependent enzyme with a molecular mass of 43 kDa and containing 354 amino acids and is classified as an aryldialkyl phosphatase [4]. Synthesis of PON1 is mainly hepatic. From liver, it is secreted into the bloodstream, where it is tightly bound to HDL particles [6]. Structurally, it is a six-bladed beta-propeller with a central tunnel containing two calcium ions—a structural one which is necessary for the conformational stability of the enzyme, and a catalytic one. Addition of EDTA (which removes calcium by complexing with it) resulted in the inactivation of paraoxon and phenyl acetate hydrolysis of PON1, showing that they are Ca^{2+}-dependent activities. However, there was no effect on the ability of PON1 to protect low density lipoprotein (LDL) from oxidation, thus implying that the antioxidant property of PON is independent of Ca^{2+} [7, 8]. This leads to the possibility of existence of different active sites on PON1 for those dependent on Ca^{2+}-dependent, and for those independent of the same, like protection against oxidation [9]. The amino terminal end of the protein contains hydrophobic amino acid residues that play a role in its binding to HDL and to other proteins such as apoA1 as well as in its self-aggregation. Recently, it has been shown that modulating the hydrophobicity of PON1 can affect organophosphatase activity of the enzyme [10].

A histidine-histidine (His) catalytic dyad is proposed to be involved in the catalytic mechanism of PON1 in which His-115 acts as a general base to deprotonate a single water molecule while His-134 increases His-115 basicity via a proton shuttle mechanism; however, some researchers found that it may participate in the substrate binding and/or orientation [11, 12]. Due to such a wide range of activities as well as being the first to be discovered, PON1 is the most studied one compared to other members. PON1 is thought to play an important role in a variety of disorders including metabolic syndrome, diabetes, atherosclerosis which results in cerebrovascular and cardiovascular events, because it is closely associated with the prevention of oxidative stress and inflammation, and is a determinant of HDL dysfunctionality. There are evidences suggestive of its atheroprotective effects through various mechanisms—maintaining cholesterol homeostasis, regulating cholesterol efflux from macrophages, as an effective xenobiotic metabolizer, and by participating in endothelial homeostasis [5, 13–16].

N-acylhomoserine γ-lactones (AHL) are produced by gram negative bacteria and regulate bacterial virulence and biofilm formation. All three PONs hydrolyse AHL with PON2 having the greatest efficacy, the resulting metabolites are inactive therefore the PON family could be important in preventing bacterial infections [17].

2. Paraoxonase 1

Oxidative stress due to reactive oxygen species results in oxidation of LDL particles and phospholipids, especially phosphatidylcholine, of the cell membrane of macrophages. This leads to a state of cellular damage and inflammation. It is possible that PON1 acts on oxidized phosphatidylcholine to produce lactone which further taken care by PON1 lactonase activity.

PON1 also exhibits homocysteine-thiolactonase activity. Homocysteine (Hcy) is a four-carbon amino acid with free thiol group formed by demethylation of methionine. Plasma Hcy levels are affected by both acquired and genetic factors [18, 19]. High levels of Hcy have been implicated in the development of cardiovascular and cerebrovascular disorders. Elevated Hcy has been shown to cause homocysteinylation, induction of oxidative stress and excitotoxicity, leading to atherosclerotic and thrombotic effects [20]. Hyperhomocysteinemia results in excess production of Homocysteine-thiolactone. This modifies proteins of coagulation, lipoproteins, endothelial receptors and is an important risk factor for adverse vascular events [21, 22]. Thus hyperhomocysteinemia, encompassing higher concentrations of homocysteine-thiolactone, may be an added risk factor for enhanced atherogenesis. PON1 has been postulated to detoxify the Hcy with its homocysteine-thiolactonase activity. At the same time, it can also protect macrophages from oxidation and prevents further inflammatory cascades. Hence the patients with low PON1 arylesterase and lactonase activity are more susceptible for the deleterious effects of lipid peroxidation, homocysteine-thiolactone toxicity and macrophage activation, which would increase the risk of neurovascular disease [23].

As a xenobiotic metabolizer, PON1 provides link between exposure to pesticides and adverse effects. The products formed by action of PON1 are considered to be the markers of pesticide exposure due to which they can be useful in the assessment of severity of pesticide exposure. Animal studies have demonstrated the potential application of PON1 in tackling the effect of pesticide poisoning. But more advanced and stringent clinical trials are required to support the definitive role in pesticide poisoning [5, 24]. PON1 response to pesticides depends upon the genetic polymorphism like Q192R, L55M. Literature reports that 192Q is more protective than 192R towards prevention of LDL oxidation.

2.1 PON1 and ischemic stroke

Globally recognized among the common causes of death, ischemic stroke accounts for major disabilities too. It is a classical multi-factorial disease with major risk factors such as hypertension, smoking, hyperlipidemia, obesity, diabetes, and atrial fibrillation. Many studies have been conducted to search for role of PON1 in ischemic stroke. Literature reports R allele and RR genotype of Q192R PON1 polymorphism carries higher risk of ischemic stroke. Many researchers have found that decrease in activity of PON1 is associated with vascular events [25, 26]. Some report, paraoxonase and arylesterase activities and their ratio can be used either to predict or to access the severity of ischemic stroke [27, 28]. In general there is significant negative correlation of PON1 activities with adverse vascular events. Lower the activities, more advanced are the vascular lesions [29, 30].

2.2 PON1 and dementias

Erstwhile dementia is now termed as major neuro-cognitive disorder (MND). It describes an overall decline in memory and cognitive skills severe enough to reduce person's ability to perform everyday activities. Previously thought to affect elderly only now it is affecting the younger age group too. It is characterized by significant decline in any of the cognitive domain including, executive function, complex attention, language, learning, memory, and perceptual-motor or social cognition. Major neuro-cognitive disorder is diagnose by the decline in patient's previous cognitive ability without delirium, which should be persistent and progressive over the time. At present disease burden supposed to be 43 million worldwide which is expected to escalate to 131 million by 2050. Alzheimer disease (AD) which is responsible for nearly 70–80% cases of dementia worldwide, is one of the important cause of death over the age of 65 years [31].

One of the characteristic neuro-pathological features of AD is the presence of amyloid plaques which comprise aggregates of β-amyloid derived from the amyloid precursor protein [32]. Increasing evidence suggests that cholesterol plays a role in the pathophysiology of Alzheimer's disease, and elevated serum total-cholesterol level has been shown to be a risk factor for AD [33]. Abnormal phosphorylation of tau proteins is thought to be responsible for pathogenesis of AD. In addition to phosphorylation, neuronal degeneration is caused by a combination of beta amyloid production, oxygen deficiency. Lipid peroxidation too plays role in pathogenesis of AD. Amyloid is responsible for oxidative stress through free radicals. This oxidative stress is responsible for conversion of soluble amyloid proteins to insoluble fibrils and further in to polymerization of tau proteins [34, 35]. Some researchers report that deficient serum paraoxonase activity is a significant risk factor for AD and that paraoxonase activity is governed in part by at least 2 distinct variants, one located in the PON1 region and another in PON2 [36]. Some reports suggest that low PON1 activity is associated with cognitive decline, especially in AD [37]. There are many opposite results regarding polymorphism In MND. Some says there is definite correlation between the Q192R and L55M polymorphism and risk of AD and MND while others differ in their views as they found no correlation [38, 39].

2.3 PON1 and Parkinson's disease

Parkinson's disease (PD) is an idiopathic disease of the nervous system characterized by both motor and non-motor system manifestations. It is a chronic progressive neurodegenerative disorder that occurs mostly in older persons but that can appear in much younger patients. It is the second most common neurodegenerative disease. Sometimes called "paralysis agitans", PD is uncommon in young people, especially those under 40 years of age [40, 41]. The pathological definition of PD is loss or degeneration of the dopaminergic neurons in the substantia nigra and development of Lewy Bodies in dopaminergic neurons. Pathologic changes may precede obvious symptoms by two decades or more. This preferential loss of dopamine producing neurons and simultaneous lack of cholinesterase inhibition results in marked imbalance acetylcholine and dopamine along with impairment of motor control. Lewy Bodies, or abnormal intracellular aggregates, contain various proteins including α-synuclein and ubiquitin that impair optimal neuron functioning [42, 43].

While the exact pathogenesis of the disease has not been completely elucidated, several theories implicating the association of genetic and environmental toxic elements such as exposure to pesticides or an oxidative cell environment conspire to trigger the neuron degeneration. Recent reports suggest that the chronic low-grade inflammation due to various sources like pesticides, drugs, aging process etc. is responsible for the cellular senescence in nervous tissue [44, 45]. From a pathologic perspective, the brain's substantia nigra pars compacta and pontine locus ceruleus are affected by typical abnormalities of PD including depigmentation, neuronal loss and gliosis. Nearly 60–70% neurons are lost by the time symptoms appears [46, 47].

Pesticides have been implicated in the development of PD by inhibition of ubiquitine proteosome system. Probably upon exposure to pesticides, mitochondrial dysfunction and α-synuclein, which is a neuronal protein, undergo conformational change which leads to symptoms of PD. One hypothesis states that as a result of mitochondrial dysfunction, there is release of cytochrome-c in the cytosol which binds to apaf1 and starts apoptosis. This results into neuronal degeneration and ultimately to PD [48].

As PON1 has antioxidant capacity and is capable of hydrolyzing toxic substances, literature links PON1 polymorphism with PD. PON1 polymorphism as Met54 may be an independent risk factor for PD. This mutation could possibly be responsible for decreased PON1 activity which results in lessened metabolism of environmental neurotoxins and could play a role in neuro-degeneration. Researchers have found that there is an association between L55M polymorphism of PON1 and PD, whereas Q192R polymorphism was unlikely to be a major risk factor for susceptibility to PD [49]. Recently a researcher found MM PON1–55 genotype exhibit greater than 2-fold increase in PD risk when exposed to organophosphates, compared with subjects who had the wild type or heterozygous genotype and no exposure [50].

2.4 PON1 and multiple sclerosis

Multiple sclerosis (MS) is one of the most common neurological disorders, occurring mainly in young adults in age 20–40 years and more commonly in women. MS is a chronic inflammatory disease characterized by demyelinating lesions in the brain, spinal cord, and optic nerve [51, 52]. Some studies have suggested a role of the oxidative stress and lipid peroxidation in the pathogenesis of MS. Due to the pathogenetic role of reactive oxygen species and the oxidation of lipoproteins in MS pathology, antioxidants prevent free-radical mediated tissue destruction [53]. PON1 is shown to play an important antioxidant role in the blood. Variability of PON1 activity depends on polymorphism in the coding region. There are only a few studies that describe the relationship between PON1 polymorphism and the risk for MS [54]. The relationship between MS and oxidative stress due to oxidized lipoproteins in cholesterol transport has been discussed. It has been proposed that increased number of oxidized HDL particles due to decreased PON activity may be unable to protect LDL against oxidation increasing the risk of atherogenesis which may lead to MS [55].

Oxidative stress is a critical factor in pathogenesis of MS as it promotes leukocyte migration, participates in oligodendrocyte damage and axonal injury. Reactive oxygen species and reactive nitrogen species are produced in the CNS of MS patients chiefly by activated macrophages and microglia could account for demyelination and axonal disruption, the hallmarks of the disease [56, 57].

2.5 PON1 and amyotrophic lateral sclerosis

Amyotrophic lateral sclerosis (ALS) is a dangerous neurodegenerative disease, characterized by progressive motor neurons loss, paralysis, and inflammation with an average survival of 3–5 years after diagnosis. 5–10% of cases are familial, and 70% of the familial cases can be explained by identified gene mutations, e.g. the *C9orf72* repeat expansion [58]. ALS is a degenerative disease of adult-onset and fatal outcome characterized by the simultaneous loss of motor neurons in the cerebral cortex, brainstem and spinal cord. In the familial cases, a large number of mutations have been found, most prominent of which is the mutation in the gene that encodes for the cytosolic enzyme superoxide dismutase [59, 60]. It was found in recent studies that PON1 gene is down-regulated in the central nervous system and peripheral cell like lymphocytes and fibroblasts. Some genetic mutations also are identified in the patients of ALS [61, 62]. It is well established fact that the oxidative stress is responsible for degeneration of the motor neurons in ALS. The CNS as a whole is particularly susceptible to oxidative stress because the neuronal membrane contains a high abundance of polyunsaturated fatty acids, especially arachidonic and docosahexaenoic acids; it consumes oxygen at a high rate; and it contains high concentrations of redox-active transition metals but a relatively low concentration of antioxidants. In ALS, at the cellular level, genetic factors, excitotoxicity, apoptosis, inflammation, mitochondrial dysfunction, protein aggregates, and oxidative stress are among the primary hypotheses put forth to explain motor neuron degeneration. Among these factors, oxidative stress appears intimately linked to a series of cellular events in motor neurons that contribute to neuronal degeneration and death [63, 64]. Individuals that had the homozygous genotypes RR and heterozygous GQ had a lower survival rate when compared to the homozygote genotype QQ. Moreover, the allele R was associated with bulbar onset. Some authors have mentioned the increased chance of ALS following the exposure to pesticides and the susceptibility increases two folds with single nucleotide polymorphisms (SNPs) like G-832A, G-162A and C-108 T [65, 66].

3. Paraoxonase 2

The PON2 isoform is highly expressed in several different types of human cells and tissues, mainly in macrophages and hepatocytes, lower lung airways, brain, cardiac and gastrointestinal systems. It is found in association with the endoplasmic reticulum and mitochondria, specifically associating with complex III of the inner mitochondrial membrane. PON2 deficiency alters mitochondrial function by decreasing mitochondrial complex I and III activity and total ATP levels and alters mitochondrial oxidative stress by increasing mitochondrial superoxide production, increasing lipid peroxidation and decreasing reduced glutathione levels. In vascular cells, PON2 has been found to be a cell-based enzyme and appeared in two glycosylated isoforms of approximately 40–43 kDa. PON2 is not detectable in plasma. In brain tissue, PON2 is an antioxidant intracellular enzyme against oxidative stress. In CNS, PON2 expression has been found in nucleus accumbens, striatum and substantia nigra. PON2 is found in astrocytes and neurons in different amounts. However, the loss of PON2 expression in both cells negatively modifies the cellular ability to recover from oxidative damage and subsequently death [67, 68].

PON2 is the oldest yet least studied variant of the paraoxonase family – its intracellular location has made studies challenging. Its three-dimensional structure has not been elucidated, nor has its intracellular compartmental distribution been determined. It has been found in multiple subcellular compartments. PON2 is highly expressed in vital organs such as the heart, brain, and the lungs, and ubiquitously found throughout the body in multiple different tissue types. It is not found in blood/plasma [69]. At mRNA level, it is enhanced in level in the liver and ubiquitous; at the protein level its occurrence is ubiquitous. It is found on the endoplasmic reticulum, in the perinuclear region, on the membrane of mitochondria, and on the plasma membrane. It is overexpressed in cancer cells. Expression in the elderly has been shown to be lower [70].

PON2 is degraded by the ubiquitin-proteasome pathway and by ADP-ribosylation. In all cell types, its expression is upregulated by Arachidonic acid, unesterified cholesterol, pomegranate juice, Antioxidants, the licorice phytoestrogen glabidrin, and atorvastatin. Its activity is decreased by glycated compounds. The two common polymorphisms found in PON2 are [71] position 147—an Ala/Gly substitution and position 311—a Ser/Cys substitution.

An apparently benign, heterozygous frameshift mutation in PON2 is present within the general population. This suggests that haploinsufficiency of PON2 is not obviously pathogenic. Thus, only after more profound loss of function than is predicted by eliminating one functional PON2 allele occurs, as in a homozygous defect, will PON2 mutants be pathogenic [72]. Plasma membrane PONs are transmembrane proteins, with the N-terminal region forming a part of the transmembrane anchoring domain on the cytoplasmic side, and C-terminal region as the extracellular catalytic site. Like PON-1, it may counteract lipid peroxidation as well as form the first line of defense for the cell against any microbial invasion [69].

PON2 has multiple enzyme functions as:

- Lactonase—hydrolyzes quorum sensing signaling molecules of bacteria. These signaling molecules, in simple terms, detect cell population density and respond to it by gene regulation. They have lactonase group in structure and are involved in autoinduction. Lactonase activity results in inhibition of these, leading to inhibition of microbial mechanisms of pathogenesis, as well as biofilm inhibition, thus forming a defense against infection, especially on the plasma membrane. Its lactonase activity has been found to be higher than PON-1 and PON-3. The Ser/Cys substitution polymorphism at position 311 affects the lactonase activity.

- Antioxidant—reduces oxidative stress in mitochondria and endoplasmic reticulum, and reduces the amount of oxidized LDLs. Deficiency of PON2, and even single nucleotide polymorphisms of the enzyme, have been shown to increase susceptibility to oxidative stress and the injury caused thereby. It is associated with mitochondrial ETC helping in sequestering ROS; however, the enzymatic nature of its overall antioxidant activity has not been proven. In endothelial cells, PON2 has been shown to reduce the production of specifically the superoxide radical but not of that of the others. Its ROS-eliminating function is probably independent of lactonase activity since the 311 Ser/Cys mutation does not affect antioxidant property and is associated with Coenzyme Q in bacteria. The exact mechanism is not understood.

It may also hydrolyze arylesters and other esters, however, unlike PON1 and PON3, its paraoxonase and statinase activities have not been detected. As said earlier, PON2 has antioxidative function, which leads to reduce oxidized LDL levels by preventing LDL oxidation and reversing the oxidation of mildly reduced LDL. This leads to inhibition of the monocyte chemotaxis associated with oxidized LDL, and increased efflux of cholesterol. Thus, PON2 is antiatherogenic.

3.1 Distribution of PON2 in the nervous system

PON2 is the only PON to be expressed in the brain. Distribution in the spinal cord has not been described adequately. Most information of the probable role of PON2 in brain is extrapolated from studies on mice [69].

PON2 is an intracellular protein [70]. It is postulated to be involved in neuro-protection by the virtue of its anti-inflammatory and antioxidant properties, and exclusive intracellular location. Measurement of its lactonase activity has been used to study the regional distribution and sex differences in mice and the findings have been extrapolated to humans. Higher levels are seen in [73].

- Females as compared to males. Oestradiol has been shown to increase PON2 expression level, since removing the ovaries of mice lead to reduction of PON2 levels. There is evidence that this occurs through activation of estrogen-α receptors. The oestrus cycle may play a role in regulating the dopamine levels; however, this not been verified [74]. Quercetin, a phytoestrogen, has been found to increase the levels of neuronal PON2 by increasing its synthesis. The functional consequences of higher expression of PON2 in females may have several ramifications, as multiple neurodegenerative diseases involve oxidative stress and neuroinflammation in their etiopathology and are divided on sex. For example, the incidence of Parkinson's disease (PD) is 90% higher in males, pointing to a protective mechanism in females that may involve PON2.

- Astrocytes as compared to neurons. PON2 has been found in the cell membranes of both of these, along with in the ER and mitochondria, but its role in the cell membrane is not known [74]. PON2 deficient neurons and astrocytes exhibit significantly higher levels of ROS when exposed to oxidative compounds H2O2 and DMNQ.

- Dopaminergic regions, where oxidative stress is higher due to dopamine metabolism. PON2 is found in the highest amount in the substantia nigra, striatum, and the nucleus accumbens. Lower levels were found in the cerebral cortex, hippocampus, brainstem and cerebellum [71]. Neurons and astrocytes in the striatum have exhibited higher susceptibility to oxidative stress than those in cerebellum in PON2 deficiency.

- Premature infants and young ones as compared to the elderly. It is postulated that the levels of high PON2 in younger ages prevent neuronal oxidative stress during the period of development of brain. The age groups who had lower presence of PON2 showed higher susceptibility to oxidative stress [70]. PON2 may also serve to regulate apoptosis or play other signaling role/–s during maturation of brain.

These differences in quantification correspond to the comparative levels of neuroprotection seen in the said groups [69]. The major mechanism by which PON2 is said to reduce oxidative neuroinflammation is by regulating mitochondrial CoQ. The mechanism is applicable in all cells PON2 is present. During transport of electrons in the electron transport chain of the inner mitochondrial membrane, CoQ accepts electrons and becomes unstable. It regains its stable form by transfer of electrons.

Most electrons are transferred to Complex III and energy is generated. However, some electrons may be transferred by CoQ to oxygen molecules when reduced CoQ comes in contact with them, given rise to reactive oxygen species. PON2 has been postulated to reduce this transfer of electrons to oxygen, thereby reduced oxidative stress and consequent neuroinflammation [70].

The role of PON2 in the cytoplasm is postulated to be different than that in the mitochondria in the nervous system; however, research on this topic is next to none [73]. Further, the role of PON2 in the endoplasmic reticula of the nerves has not been studied [69]. In the brain, the loss of PON2 in both neurons and astrocytes impairs their ability to recover from toxic levels of oxidative stress generated by oxidants hydrogen peroxide (H2O2) or 2,3-dimethoxy-1,4-naphthoquinone (DMNQ) [73].

3.2 Modulation of PON2

Quercetin has been found to increase the levels of astrocyte PON2 in mice approximately two times. It is postulated that since quercetin is a phytoestrogen, it may activate estrogen-α receptors like oestradiol, leading to increased PON2 synthesis. Alternatively, the JNK/AP-1 pathway has also been suggested to be the central underlying mechanism—it was shown that inhibition of this pathway lead to antagonization of the effect of quercetin on PON2 levels [71].

3.3 Impact on motor behavior

Mice deficient in PON2 showed slightly more activity during the dark cycle than mice having PON2. There were no differences in food consumption. During the rotarod experiment, PON2 deficient mice had significant shorter latency to fall, suggesting impaired motor co-ordination [73].

3.4 Probable role in dopaminergic system

Oxidation of dopamine during its metabolism generates free radicals and reactive quinones in the dopaminergic neurons. Due to this additional oxidative burden, the dopaminergic neurons are more susceptible to additional oxidative stress, neuroinflammation and cellular death. PON2 reduces the oxidative stress here by inhibition of superoxide formation by mitochondrial CoQ [74]. PON2 was also found to be modulated by dopamine receptor activity in a receptor-specific manner, with protein and transcript upregulated in neurons upon exposure to a dopamine receptor 2 agonist, but not an agonist for dopamine receptor 1 [73].

PON2 has been shown to interact with PARK7 in vivo. The protective antioxidant effects of PARK7 are partly mediated by expression of PON2 [74]. *In vitro*, PON2 has been shown to reduce the increased susceptibility of striatal neurons to oxidative stress in cases of PARK7 deficiency [73].

In mice, in PON2 deficient striatum, the levels of tyrosine hydroxylase protein were found to be lower and that of tyrosine hydroxylase transcript were found to be higher than in the wild type (with PON2 present). The levels of Vesicular Amine Transporter 2 (VMAT2) transcript were found to be increased but there was no change in protein levels. The levels of Dopamine Transporter, which is involved in the reuptake of dopamine form the synaptic cleft, were found to be unchanged at both the transcript and protein level. Dopamine receptors DRD-1, DRD-2, and DRD-5 were found to be upregulated at the transcript level but not at the protein level in PON2 deficiency. Thus, PON2 deficiency significantly upregulates the transcript of multiple dopaminergic related genes in the striatum of mice.

Transcript levels of antioxidant enzymes, heme-oxygeneases-1 and -2 and MADPH-oxidase 2, were increased in PON2 deficient mice, although the protein levels were not altered. This implied that in absence of PON2, the oxidative stress in these neurons increased, due to which levels of antioxidant enzymes were increased [74].

3.5 PON2 and Parkinson disease

As said above, PON2 interacts with the DJ-1 (PARK7) gene. Of all cases of familial Parkinson's disease (PD), loss-of-function mutations in DJ-1 (PARK7) gene account for about 1%. The actions of this gene are said to reduce the oxidative stress-mediated damage; however, the mechanisms for the same are unknown. It was shown that *in vivo*, PON2 associates with DJ-1.

MPTP is one of the causative agents of Parkinson Disease, and it, along with its metabolite MPP is used for research regarding Parkinson disease. MPP is a complex I inhibitor which leads to oxidative stress and death of a number of different neurons. Exposure to MPP lead to increase in the PON2 lactonase activity in mice. It was found that in deficiency of DJ-1 both the basal and MPP-induced lactonase activity of PON2 was blocked. Loss of DJ-1 thus impairs PON2 activity. However, it was also noted that DJ-1 does not alter PON2 levels in neurons, implying that it increases PON2 activity by increasing the rate of enzyme action, and not the amount of enzyme synthesized. The exact mechanism is unclear.

Absence of either of PON2 or DJ-1 leads to increased sensitivity of the neuron towards oxidative stress by MPP. Interestingly, PON2 expression effectively rescues DJ-1 deficiency-mediated hypersensitivity to oxidative stress, although DJ-1 expression cannot do so for PON2. This suggests PON2 to be a downstream target of DJ-1. Thus, PON2 expression protects neurons against MPP and can also reverse the hypersensitivity observed with DJ-1 loss [75].

3.6 PON2 and amyotrophic lateral sclerosis

ALS is a neurodegenerative disorder of spinal tract. It is a multifactorial disease characterized by cerebral cell dysfunction and mitochondrial alteration. It is associated with the progressive increase in neuro-inflammation, generalized oxidative stress and metabolic alterations. The C allele of the C311S PON2 has been associated with sporadic ALS. In addition, the expression of messenger RNA of the PON2 gene was decreased in spinal cord and trunk tissue of patients with ALS [76]. ALS-associated variant in PON2 is present as a homozygous defect.

However, since there are multiple substrates for PONs, it is difficult to ascertain the exact role of PONs in the pathogenesis of AML. ALS-related mutations have been found in all the three forms of PON, implying a higher probability that the property of the PONs which plays a role in pathogenesis is likely to be a common property/feature. One of the theories says that loss of antioxidant functions of the PONs leads to the inability of nervous tissue to detoxify the abnormal oxidative stresses the motor neurons and spinal cord are exposed to, leading to neurotoxicity. Another theory says that mutations in PONs may lead to failure to inhibit some unknown exotoxin, which leads to ALS [72].

3.7 PON2 and glioblastoma

In all cancers, PON2 is overexpressed. Due to its antioxidant effect, PON-2 reduces cellular oxidative damage and influences redox signaling, which promotes cellular survival [70]. PON2 in tumor cells probably protects the intracellular membranes against oxidation and, possibly, prevents free radicals from percolating through the nuclear envelope and damaging the genetic material contained in the cells [74]. Elevated PON-2 levels may stabilize tumor cells by enhancing cellular stress resistance, attenuating mitochondrial ROS-mediated apoptosis [70].

The highest expression of PON2 is observed in liver and brain cancers. PON2 was localized in the perinuclear region. In glioblastoma, PON2 gene is amplified. The level of PON2 was a negative prognostic factor in glioblastoma [77]. Valproic acid has been shown to inhibit the growth of glioblastoma and increase the production of reactive oxygen species in glioblastoma cells. This was attributed to inhibition of PON2 by valproic acid at the transcriptional level. This deceased PON2 expression could potentiate the cytotoxic effects of ROS and enhance VPA-induced cell cycle arrest. The use of the model of transfectants overexpressing PON2 provided further support for VPA-induced GBM cell growth suppression being mediated by increased ROS production and that the effect was augmented by decreased PON2 [78].

3.8 Developmental expression of PON2

In mice, PON2 protein appears to be lowest directly after birth, steadily increasing with age up until Post-natal Day (PND) 21. A significant decrease in both protein and mRNA is noted from PND 21 to 30 and continuing to PND 60. In monkeys, PON2 protein levels were lower at mid-gestation and gradually increased up to infant age. This was followed by a decrease in the juvenile stage and a stabilization, in which similar levels were found in young adult and in aged monkey brains. The overall trend observed in both species reveals a possible window of susceptibility to oxidative stress in young adult mice and monkeys which may point to a change in cellular environment driving a decrease in PON2 expression [73].

3.9 PON2 and age

Expression of PON2 decreases with age. Thus, with growing age, the susceptibility to oxidative damage is increased, in turn increasing the risk for neurodegenerative diseases. In mice, concurrent to PON2 deficiency, transcripts of glucose transporter 4, insulin receptor and tau were upregulated, while butyrylcholinesterase was significantly downregulated, potentially having neurodegenerative consequences. However, the findings supported a lack of oxidative stress in the aged brain with potential impacts to endogenous signaling and host immunity through a reduction in cytokine expression [73].

3.10 PON2 and future perspectives

The identification and initial characterization of PON2 in brain tissue suggest that this enzyme may play a relevant role in determining susceptibility to oxidative stress and neuroinflammation, and that its positive modulation may represent a novel strategy for neuroprotection. Attempts to elevate PON2 levels could be neuroprotective. For tumor cells, PON2 overexpression probably provides resistance of these cells to apoptosis and that a useful therapeutic strategy would be one causing a decrease of PON2 [71].

4. Paraoxonase 3

PON3 is an antioxidant hydrolase enzyme with approximately 40-kDa, synthesized in the liver. In plasma PON3 is bound to HDL and apolipoprotein—A1 and possesses strong anti-oxidant properties but its concentration is about two orders of magnitude less abundant than PON1. PON3 is also expressed at low levels in the kidney. PON3 was the last enzyme in the paraoxonase family genetic cluster to be described. Currently, very little is known about its function and physiological characteristics in humans. The enzymes PON3 and PON1 show some similarities in structure and hydrolase activity. Regarding the structure, both enzymes have three highly conserved cysteine (Cys) residues in positions -41; -283 and -351 in the protein chain. As for enzyme activity, PON3 can hydrolyze cyclic carbonate esters and lactones rapidly, mainly drugs such as statin lactones. The arylesterase activity of PON3 is almost undetectable when compared to PON1 [79, 80].

PON3 protein expression in the white-matter brain areas of healthy C57BL/6J mice. One study reports that there is strong evidence of PON1 and PON3 expression surrounding Aβ plaques, and intense positive staining in star-shaped cells that resembled glial cells in areas with an abundance of Aβ plaques [81]. It was suggested in the study that localization of PON1 and PON3 in astrocytes or oligodendrocytes, at the same time there is colocalization of PON3 in microglia which indicates a potential antioxidant role of PON1 and PON3 in decreasing levels of ROS and/or preventing lipid peroxidation in these cells in Alzheimer disease pathology.

Although there is no documented *PON1* or *PON3* gene expression in any of the mouse- or human-brain regions, one of the study indicated that PON1 and PON3 proteins are expressed in myelinated fibers in the brain tissue of healthy C57BL/6 mice. This suggests that PON1 and PON3 are somehow transferred from blood circulation to the brain [82]. Overall the PON3 is much less studied as compared to PON1 & PON2. So much less information is available in the literature than others.

4.1 Paraoxonases and acetylcholine esterase

PON1 and Acetylcholine esterase are both serum ester hydrolases. Genes for both are located on the same chromosome—7q1-22—near to each other [83]. At the genetic level, due to the proximity in their locations, it is thought that the genes for both would be regulated by a locus control region. It has been shown that PON1 and acetylcholinesterase share an inverse relationship. This relationship is not shown by pseudocholinesterase. It is thought that the same locus control region may control their interactions. Acetylcholine esterase is especially susceptible to oxidative stress, and paraoxonase is an antioxidant. This also contributes to their interactions.

Organophosphates are inhibitors of acetylcholine esterase (AChE). They are metabolized in liver to form oxones, which irreversibly inhibit AChE. The usual form of AChE is oligomeric and it is this form which is inhibited by organophosphate compounds (OPCs). On inhibition, up-regulation at genetic level causes increase in synthesis of AChE; however, this AChE is unable to oligomerize. This form of AChE, also called $AChE_R$, is thought to act in inflammatory processes, contributing to the disease pathobiology. PON1 is a key detoxifier of organophosphates and organophosphate exposure has been linked to the development of neurological disorders where acetylcholine plays a significant role [84].

PON1 is thought to protect AChE through its antioxidant action by neutralizing superoxide radicals. They also spare AChE from organophosphates by lysis of organophosphate compounds. Exposure to OPCs usually results from chronic domestic pesticide exposure. PON1 polymorphisms result in hypofunction of PON1. In such states, OPCs irreversibly inactivate circulating AChE. PON1 usually is not a vital enzyme, but in case of a person with PON1 polymorphism, exposure to OPCs may trigger detrimental effects of the polymorphism present. In absence of functional PON1, the organophosphate exposure results in irreversible inhibition of the circulating oligomeric AChE and up-regulation of $AChE_R$. Thus, presence of PON1 is thought to prevent this by its antioxidant and paraoxonase activities, and genetic variations in PON1 affect the individual's susceptibility to OPC exposure [85].

The nigrostriatal pathway of dopamine secretion degenerates with increasing age. This leads to minor DA depletion. In people with intact and functional AChE and PON1, this minor depletion does not cause any significant detrimental alteration in health, even in presence of OPCs exposure. However, in presence of polymorphisms in either of AChE or PON1, this can predispose to Parkinson disease. In Parkinson disease, the acetylcholine and dopamine levels are imbalanced with respect to each other due to damage to the substantia nigra. Chronic exposure to OPCs aggravates this imbalance by the means explained above. PON1 counters this imbalance through its antioxidant and paraoxonase activities [84].

Alzheimer disease, on the other hand, is linked to cholinergic deficiency. Hence, AChE inhibitors (AChEIs) are used to treat it. However, the response of patients to these AChEIs is not uniform—many patients have been found not to respond to the same. It was discovered that the AChEI activity was inversely related to PON2 esterase activity. Further investigations [85] revealed that this was most likely because the esterase activity of PON2 lead to the lysis of the AChEIs. While PON1 mutations did not have this esterase effect on these drugs, the PON2 polymorphic forms, 311C and 148G, showed increased esterase activity. Thus, PON2 analysis in patients with Alzheimer disease may indicate whether the AChEI therapy would be successful or not [86].

We can conclude that the paraoxonase is the molecule which has implications in the neurodegenerative disease and other aspects of nervous system. Mostly the role of paraoxonase is protective one by the virtue of prevention of oxidative stress which arises due to the imbalance in the redox system. But this is only the tip off the iceberg as more research is required in this aspect.

Author details

Mohit Vijay Rojekar[1]*, Kaushalraj Sunil Dandegonker[1] and Swati Ghanghurde[2]

1 Department of Biochemistry, Rajiv Gandhi Medical College, Thane, India

2 Department of Pathology, Rajiv Gandhi Medical College, Thane, India

*Address all correspondence to: drmohi44@gmail.com

References

[1] La Du BN. Structural and functional diversity of paraoxonases. Nature Medicine. 1996;**2**(11):1186-1187

[2] Mikhail MS, Anyaegbunam A, Garfinkel D, Palan PR, Basu J, Romney SL. Preeclampsia and antioxidant nutrients: Decreased plasma levels of reduced ascorbic acid, alpha-tocopherol, and beta-carotene in women with preeclampsia. American Journal of Obstetrics and Gynecology. 1994;**171**(1):150-157

[3] Mackness MI, Mackness B, Durrington PN, Connelly PW, Hegele RA. Paraoxonase: Biochemistry, genetics and relationship to plasma lipoproteins. Current Opinion in Lipidology. 1996;7(2):69-76

[4] Mackness M, Mackness B. Human paraoxonase-1 (PON1): Gene structure and expression, promiscuous activities and multiple physiological roles. Gene. 2015;**567**:12-21

[5] Costa LG, Giordano G, Cole TB, Marsillach J, Furlong CE. Paraoxonase 1 (PON1) as a genetic determinant of susceptibility to organophosphate toxicity. Toxicology. 2013;**307**:115-122

[6] Deakin S, Leviev I, Gomaraschi M, Calabresi L, Francesshini G, James RW. Enzymatically active paraoxonase-1 is located at the external membrane of producing cells and released by a high affinity, saturable, desorption mechanism. The Journal of Biological Chemistry. 2002;**277**:4301-4308

[7] Harel M, Aharoni A, Gaidukov L, Brumshtein B, Khersonsky O, Meged R, et al. Structure and evolution of the serum paraoxonase family of detoxifying and anti- atherosclerotic enzymes. Nature Structural & Molecular Biology. 2004;**11**:412

[8] Blaha-Nelson D, Krüger DM, Szeler K, Ben-David M, Kamerlin SCL. Active site hydrophobicity and the convergent evolution of paraoxonase activity in structurally divergent enzymes: The case of serum paraoxonase 1. Journal of the American Chemical Society. 2017;**139**:1155-1167

[9] Aviram M, Billecke S, Sorenson R, Bisgaier C, Newton R, Rosenblat M, et al. Paraoxonase active site required for protection against LDL oxidation involves its free sulfhydryl group and is different from that required for its arylesterase/ paraoxonase activities: Selective action of human paraoxonase allozymes Q and R. Arteriosclerosis, Thrombosis, and Vascular Biology. 1998;**18**:1617-1624

[10] Sorenson RC, Primo-Parmo SL, Kuo CL, Adkins S, Lockridge O, La Du BN. Reconsideration of the catalytic center and mechanism of mammalian paraoxonase/arylesterase. Proceedings of the National Academy Science USA. 1995;**92**:7187-7191

[11] Khersonsky O, Tawfik DS. Structure-reactivity studies of serum paraoxonase PON1 suggest that its true native activity is lactonase. Biochemistry. 2005;**44**:6371-6382

[12] Grunkemeyer TJ, Mata DG, Doddapaneni K, Murali S, Magliery TJ. Insights into the mechanism of paraoxonase-1: Comparing the reactivity of the six-bladed β-propeller hydrolases. Biochemistry. 2018:1-46

[13] Adhe-Rojekar A, Mogarekar MR, Rojekar MV. Study of serum Paraoxonase and high density lipoprotein fractions in

diabetes. Iranian Journal of Diabetes and Obesity. 2018;**10**(1):16-22

[14] Rojekar M, Mogarekar M, Adhe-Rojekar A. Study of oxidative stress marker serum paraoxonase in metabolic syndrome. Turkish Journal of Endocrinology & Metabolism. 2016;**20**(3):83-87

[15] James RW. A long and winding road: Defining the biological role and clinical importance of paraoxonases. Clinical Chemistry and Laboratory Medicine. 2006;**44**:1052-1059

[16] Berrougui H, Loued S, Khalil A. Purified human paraoxonase-1 interacts with plasma membrane lipid rafts and mediates cholesterol efflux from macrophages. Free Radical Biology & Medicine. 2012;**52**:1372-1381

[17] Teiber JF, Horke S, Haines DC, Chowdhary PK, Xiao J, Kramer GL, et al. Dominant role of paraoxonases in inactivation of the Pseudomonas aeruginosa quorum- sensing signal N-(3-oxododecanoyl)-L-homoserine lactone. Infection and Immunity. 2008;**76**:2512-2519

[18] Kluijtmans LA, Young IS, Boreham CA, Murray L, McMaster D, McNulty H, et al. Genetic and nutritional factors contributing to hyperhomocysteinemia in young adults. Blood. 2003;**101**(7):2483-2488

[19] Dierkes J, Westphal S. Effect of drugs on homocysteine concentrations. Seminars in Vascular Medicine. 2005;**5**(2):124-139

[20] Škovierová H, Vidomanová E, Mahmood S, Sopková J, Drgová A, Červeňová T, et al. The molecular and cellular effect of homocysteine metabolism imbalance on human health. International Journal of Molecular Sciences. 2016;**17**(10):1733

[21] Aviram M. Review of human studies on oxidative damage and antioxidant protection related to cardiovascular diseases. Free Radical Research. 2000;**33**(Suppl):S85-S97

[22] Mackness M, Mackness B. Targeting paraoxonase-1 in atherosclerosis. Expert Opinion on Therapeutic Targets. 2013;**17**:829-837

[23] Richter RJ, Jarvik GP, Furlong CE. Paraoxonase 1 (PON1) status and substrate hydrolysis. Toxicology and Applied Pharmacology. 2009;**235**:1-9

[24] Furlong CE, Suzuki SM, Stevens RC, et al. Human PON1, a biomarker of risk of disease and exposure. Chemico-Biological Interactions. 2010;**187**:355-361

[25] Liu H, Xia P, Liu M, et al. PON gene polymorphisms and ischaemic stroke: A systematic review and meta analysis. International Journal of Stroke. 2013;**8**:111-123

[26] Mahrooz A, Gohari G, Hashemi MB, et al. R-carrying genotypes of serum paraoxonase (PON1) 192 polymorphism and higher activity ratio are related to susceptibility against ischemic stroke. Molecular Biological Reports. 2012;**39**:11177-11185

[27] Sand PG. Paraoxonase genes and the susceptibilty to ischemic stroke. International Journal of Stroke. 2013;**8**:E39

[28] Michalak S, Kazmierski R, Hellmann A, et al. Serum paraoxonase/ arylesterase activity affects outcome in ischemic stroke patients. Cerebrovascular Diseases. 2011;**32**:124-132

[29] Tang WH, Hartiala J, Fan Y, et al. Clinical and genetic association of serum paraoxonase and arylesterase activities with cardiovascular risk.

Arteriosclerosis, Thrombosis, and Vascular Biology. 2012;**32**:2803-2812

[30] Aviram M, Vaya J. Paraoxonase 1 activities, regulation, and interactions with atherosclerotic lesion. Current Opinion in Lipidology. 2013;**4**:339-344

[31] Emmady PD, Schoo C, Tadi. Major Neurocognitive Disorder (Dementia). Treasure Island (FL): StatPearls Publishing; 2022. Available from: https://www.ncbi.nlm.nih.gov/books/NBK557444/ Accessed on 01/03/2023

[32] Chartier-Harlin MC, Crawford F, Houlden H, Warren A, Hughes D, Fidani L, et al. Early-onset Alzheimer's disease caused by mutations at codon 717 of the β-amyloid precursor protein gene. Nature. 1991;**353**:844-846

[33] Kivipelto M, Helkala EL, Laakso MP, Haninnen T, Hallikainen M, Alhainen K, et al. Midlife vascular risk factors and Alzheimer's disease in later life: Longitudinal, population based study. BMJ. 2001;**322**:1447-1451

[34] Dyrks T, Dyrks E. Amyloidogenicity of beta A amyloid. The Journal of Biological Chemistry. 1992;**267**:18210-18217

[35] Troncoso J, Costello A, Watson AL Jr. In vitro polymerization of oxidized TAU into filaments. Brain Research. 1993;**613**:313-316

[36] Erlich PM, Lunetta KL, Cupples LA, Abraham CR, Green RC, Baldwin CT, et al. Serum paraoxonase activity is associated with variants in the PON gene cluster and risk of Alzheimer disease. Neurobiology of Aging. 2012;**33**(5):1015.e7-1015.23

[37] Perła-Kaján J, Włoczkowska O, Zioła-Frankowska A, Frankowski M, Smith AD, de Jager CA, et al. Paraoxonase 1, B vitamins supplementation, and mild cognitive impairment. Journal of Alzheimer's Disease. 2021;**81**(3):1211-1229

[38] Pi Y, Zhang L, Chang K, et al. Lack of an association between Paraoxonase 1 gene polymorphisms (Q192R, L55M) and Alzheimer's disease: A meta-analysis. Neuroscience Letters. 2012;**523**:174-179

[39] He XM, Zhang ZX, Zhang JW, et al. Gln192Arg polymorphism in paraoxonase 1 gene is associated with Alzheimer disease in a Chinese Han ethnic population. Chinese Medical Journal. 2006;**119**:1204-1209

[40] Sherer TB, Chowdhury S, Peabody K, Brooks D. Overcoming obstacles in Parkinson's disease. Movement Disorders. 2012;**27**(13):1606-1611

[41] Chou K. Clinical manifestations of Parkinson disease. UpToDate. 2013. Available from: www.uptodate.com [Accessed: 22 July, 2013]

[42] MacPhee G. D Stewart: Parkinson's disease. Reviews in Clinical Gerontology. 2001;**11**:33-49

[43] Gazewood J, Richards D, Clebak K. Parkinson disease: An update. American Family Physician. 2013;**87**(4):267-273

[44] Chinta S, Lieu C, Demaria M, Laberge R, Campisi J, Anderson J. Environmental stress, ageing, and glial cell senescence: A novel mechanistic link to Parkinson's disease? Journal of Internal Medicine. 2013;**273**:429-436

[45] Brown T, Rumsby P, Capleton A, Rushton L, Levy L. Pesticides and Parkinson's disease: Is there a link? Environmental Health Perspectives. 2006;**14**(2):156-164

[46] Jankovic J, Hurtig H, Dashe J. Etiology and Pathogenesis of Parkinson

Disease. UpToDate. 2013. Available from: www.uptodate.com [Accessed: 22 July, 2013]

[47] Postuma R, Gagnon J, Montplaisir J. Clinical prediction of Parkinson's disease: Planning for the age of neuroprotection. Journal of Neurology. 2009;**81**:1008-1013

[48] Camilleri A, Vassallo N. The centrality of mitochondria in the pathogenesis and treatment of Parkinson's disease. CNS Neuroscience & Therapeutics. 2014;**20**(7):591-602

[49] Zintzaras E, Hadjigeorgiou GM. Association of paraoxonase 1 gene polymorphisms with risk of Parkinson's disease: A meta-analysis. Journal of Human Genetics. 2004;**49**(9):474-481

[50] Manthripragada AD, Costello S, Cockburn MG, Bronstein JM, Ritz B. Paraoxonase 1, agricultural organophosphate exposure, and Parkinson disease. Epidemiology. 2010;**21**:87-94

[51] Nessler S, Brück W. Advances in multiple sclerosis research in 2009. Journal of Neurology. 2010;**257**(9):1590-1593

[52] Sluder JA, Newhouse P, Fain D. Pediatric and adolescent multiple sclerosis. Adolescent Medicine Clinics. 2002;**13**(3):461

[53] LeVine SM. The role of reactive oxygen species in the pathogenesis of multiple sclerosis. Medical Hypotheses. 1992;**39**(3):271-274

[54] Humbert R, Adler DA, Disteche CM, Hassett C, Omiecinski CJ, Furlong CE. The molecular basis of the human serum paraoxonase activity polymorphism. Nature Genetics. 1993;**3**(1):73-76

[55] Imai Y, Morita H, Kurihara H, Sugiyama T, Kato N, Ebihara A, et al. Evidence for association between paraoxonase gene polymorphisms and atherosclerotic diseases. Atherosclerosis. 2000;**149**(2):435-442

[56] Katz Sand IB, Lublin FD. Diagnosis and differential diagnosis of multiple sclerosis. Continuum. 2013;**19**:922-943

[57] Miller E, Wachowicz B, Majsterek I. Advances in antioxidative therapy of multiple sclerosis. Current Medicinal Chemistry. 2013;**20**(37):4720-4730

[58] DeJesus-Hernandez M, Mackenzie IR, Boeve BF, Boxer AL, Baker M, Rutherford NJ, et al. Expanded GGGGCC hexanucleotide repeat in noncoding region of C9ORF72 causes chromosome 9p-linked FTD and ALS. Neuron. 2011;**72**(2):245-256

[59] Kruger D. Amyotrophic lateral sclerosis. JAAPA. 2012;**25**:53-54

[60] Ludolph AC, Brettschneider J, Weishaupt JH. Amyotrophic lateral sclerosis. Current Opinion in Neurology. 2012;**25**:530-535

[61] Gagliardi S, Abel K, Bianchi M, Milani P, Bernuzzi S, Corato M, et al. Regulation of FMO and PON detoxication systems in ALS human tissues. Neurotoxicity Research. 2013;**23**(4):370-377

[62] Cronin S, Greenway MJ, Prehn JH, Hardiman O. Paraoxonase promoter and intronic variants modify risk of sporadic amyotrophic lateral sclerosis. Journal of Neurology, Neurosurgery, and Psychiatry. 2007;**78**:984-986

[63] Cosgrove JP, Church DF, Pryor WA. The kinetics of the autoxidation of polyunsaturated fatty acids. Lipids. 1987;**22**(5):299-304

[64] Barber SC, Shaw PJ. Oxidative stress in ALS: Key role in motor neuron injury

and therapeutic target. Free Radical Biology & Medicine. 2010;**48**(5):629-641

[65] Verde F, Tiloca C, Morelli C, Doretti A, Poletti B, Maderna L, et al. PON1 is a disease modifier gene in amyotrophic lateral sclerosis: Association of the Q192R polymorphism with bulbar onset and reduced survival. Neurological Sciences. 2019;**2019**:1469-1473

[66] Morahan JM, Yu B, Trent RJ, Pamphlett R. A gene-environment study of the paraoxonase 1 gene and pesticides in amyotrophic lateral sclerosis. Neurotoxicology. 2007;**28**:532-540

[67] Garrick JM, Dao K, de Laat R, Elsworth J, Cole TB, Marsillach J, et al. Developmental expression of paraoxonase 2. Chemico-Biological Interactions. 2016;**259**:168-174

[68] Giordano G, Cole TB, Furlong CE, Costa LG. Paraoxonase 2 (PON2) in the mouse central nervous system: A neuroprotective role? Toxicology and Applied Pharmacology. 2011;**256**:369-378

[69] Manco G, Porzio E, Carusone TM. Human paraoxonase-2 (PON2): Protein functions and modulation. Antioxidants. 2021;**10**(2):256

[70] Parween F, Gupta RD. Insights into the role of paraoxonase 2 in human pathophysiology. Journal of Biosciences. 2022;**47**(1):1-20

[71] Costa LG, de Laat R, Dao K, Pellacani C, Cole TB, Furlong CE. Paraoxonase-2 (PON2) in brain and its potential role in neuroprotection. Neurotoxicology. 2014;**43**:3-9

[72] Ticozzi N, LeClerc AL, Keagle PJ, Glass JD, Wills AM, Van Blitterswijk M, et al. Paraoxonase gene mutations in amyotrophic lateral sclerosis. Annals of Neurology. 2010;**68**(1):102-107

[73] Garrick JM. Characterizing the Role of Paraoxonase 2 (PON2) in the Brain: Phenotypic Analysis and Modulating Factors. Washington DC: University of Washington; 2021

[74] Garrick JM, Dao K, Costa LG, Marsillach J, Furlong CE. Examining the role of paraoxonase 2 in the dopaminergic system of the mouse brain. BMC Neuroscience. 2022;**23**(1):1-4

[75] Parsanejad M, Bourquard N, Qu D, Zhang Y, Huang E, Rousseaux MW, et al. DJ-1 interacts with and regulates paraoxonase-2, an enzyme critical for neuronal survival in response to oxidative stress. PLoS One. 2014;**9**(9):e106601

[76] Reichert CO, Levy D, Bydlowski SP. Paraoxonase role in human neurodegenerative diseases. Antioxidants. 2020;**10**(1):11

[77] Shakhparonov MI, Antipova NV, Shender VO, Shnaider PV, Arapidi GP, Pestov NB, et al. Expression and intracellular localization of paraoxonase 2 in different types of malignancies. Acta Naturae. 2018;**10**(3):92-99

[78] Tseng JH, Chen CY, Chen PC, Hsiao SH, Fan CC, Liang YC, et al. Valproic acid inhibits glioblastoma multiforme cell growth via paraoxonase 2 expression. Oncotarget. 2017;**8**(9):14666

[79] Lu H, Zhu J, Zang Y, Ze Y, Qin J. Cloning, high level expression of human paraoxonase-3 in Sf9 cells and pharmacological characterization of its product. Biochemical Pharmacology. 2005;**70**:1019-1025

[80] Zhou H, Zhou J, Li H, Hui C, Bi J. Paraoxonase 3 gene polymorphisms are associated with occupational noise-induced deafness: A matched

case-control study from China. PLoS One. 2020;**15**:e0240615

[81] Salazar JG, Marsillach J, Reverte I, Mackness B, Mackness M, Joven J, et al. Paraoxonase-1 and -3 protein expression in the brain of the Tg2576 mouse model of Alzheimer's disease. Antioxidants (Basel). 2021;**10**(3):339

[82] Marsillach J, Mackness B, Mackness M, Riu F, Beltrán R, Joven J, et al. Immunohistochemical analysis of Paraoxonases-1, 2, and 3 expression in Normal mouse tissues. Free Radical Biology & Medicine. 2008;**45**:146-157

[83] Fuhrman B, Partoush A, Aviram M. Acetylcholine esterase protects LDL against oxidation. Biochemical and Biophysical Research Communications. 2004;**322**(3):974-978

[84] Menini T, Gugliucci A. Paraoxonase 1 in neurological disorders. Redox Report. 2014;**19**(2):49-58

[85] Bryk B, BenMoyal-Segal L, Podoly E, Livnah O, Eisenkraft A, Luria S, et al. Inherited and acquired interactions between ACHE and PON1 polymorphisms modulate plasma acetylcholinesterase and paraoxonase activities. Journal of Neurochemistry. 2005;**92**(5):1216-1227

[86] Parween F, Hossain MS, Singh KP, Gupta RD. Association between human paraoxonase 2 protein and efficacy of acetylcholinesterase inhibiting drugs used against Alzheimer's disease. PLoS One. 2021;**16**(10):e0258879

Chapter 7

Neurotoxin Decontamination

Dongmei Ye and Susan Rempe

Abstract

Nerve agents are a group of organophosphorus (OP) compounds that are potent neurotoxins used as chemical warfare agents and insecticides. Current medical countermeasures, including atropine and oxime-based reactivators, target the down-stream pathways inhibited by OP agents and cannot effectively eliminate OP agents. In contrast, organophosphorus hydrolase (OPH) is a bacterial enzyme that can detoxify a wide range of OP agents. The advantage of OPH over oxime-based treatment is rapid hydrolysis of these agents in the circulatory system. Kinetic properties of OPH from various bacteria have been studied by others. Substrate binding affinity ranges between 200 μM and 2.5 mM, well above lethal levels. To improve OPH mutant screening capability, we optimized a cell-free protein synthesis system to express active OPH variants rapidly and conduct kinetic measurements. We also tested the hypothesis that active site mutations using only natural amino acids restrict the development of OPH variants with binding affinities close to nerve agent lethal levels (a few μM). Our work resulted in a suite of OPH variants that incorporated selected unnatural amino acids into OPH, with mutations targeted for the first time to both active and allosteric binding sites. Kinetic studies of those mutants show significantly improved OPH substrate binding affinity.

Keywords: organophosphorus hydrolase, nerve agent, paraoxon, substrate binding affinity, unnatural amino acid substitution

1. Introduction

As a neurotransmitter, acetylcholine (ACh) plays a vital role in brain and muscle function. Its function can be both excitatory and inhibitory. But in the central nervous system (CNS), ACh primarily plays the excitatory role, which means it can speed up nerve signals. Excess ACh is degraded by acetylcholinesterase (AChE) to maintain a balanced ACh level. Nerve agents are a group of organophosphorus (OP) compounds that are potent neurotoxins used as chemical warfare agents and insecticides. OP nerve agents disrupt the CNS by inhibiting AChE function. Inhibition of AChE results in ACh accumulation and ACh receptor overstimulation, leading to severe injuries and even death due to losing control of respiratory muscles. Those injured by nerve agents often express chronic health problems, such as visual impairment, dermatological conditions, neurological sequelae, and respiratory problems [1].

Weapons of mass destruction were first used in World War I. Rapid advances in chemistry during that time brought surging knowledge and constant growth in developing more effective chemical agents. The nerve agent, tabun, was first discovered from an organophosphorus insecticide in 1936 by a German chemist, Dr. Gerhart Schrader. About two years later, Dr. Schrader developed another similar nerve agent, sarin [2]. Suitable delivery systems and large-scale production of nerve agents were also developed rapidly for their usage in warfare. Since nerve agents are stable, easily dispersed and work at low concentrations, the effects are long-lasting and increase with continued exposure. The threat from nerve agents was not confined to military battlefields. The Matsumoto sarin attack (1994) and Tokyo subway sarin attack (1995) exhibited the usage of nerve agents in terrorist attacks. Paraoxon, which is the active metabolite of the insecticide parathion, is also a potent nerve agent. As such, nerve agents pose a threat to armed forces, agricultural workers, and civilians.

Current medical countermeasures available include atropine and pralidoxime chloride (2-PAM Cl). Atropine competitively inhibits ACh binding to acetylcholine receptors, reducing receptor overstimulation. The therapeutic 2-PAM Cl re-cleaves AChE phosphorylation induced by nerve agents and reactivates AChE. These countermeasures target the down-stream pathways of OP; thus, none of them effectively eliminates OP agents.

A direct method that can hydrolyze OP agents before they enter the central nervous system is urgently needed. Organophosphorus hydrolase (OPH) is a bacterial enzyme that can detoxify a wide range of OP nerve agents and pesticides. The advantage of OPH over existing treatments is rapid hydrolysis of OP agents, which provides the potential to eliminate nerve agents in the circulatory system, before they penetrate the blood-brain barrier and exert effects in the CNS. Kinetic properties of OPH from various bacteria have been studied, with k_{cat} about 10^3/s–10^4/s and K_m between 80 μM and 2.5 mM [3, 4], significantly higher compared to nerve agent lethal levels (a few μM).

The OPH active site is dominated by histidine residues and stabilized by the stacking network formed among these histidine residues. This unique feature makes OPH a great candidate for aromatic unnatural amino acid (UAA) substitutions. In this chapter, we first describe a high-throughput cell-free protein synthesis and kinetic measurement method for rapid screening and selection of OPH variants with enhanced substrate binding. Then, we examine the possibility to apply cell-free protein synthesis systems for expression of OPH UAA substitutions. Lastly, we present a genetic code expansion (GCE) machinery used to examine the expression of OPH UAA substitutions. The results of kinetic studies of these mutants showed greatly improved OPH substrate binding affinity. Overall, this work uniquely demonstrates that UAA replacements can enhance enzyme properties significantly.

2. Bio-engineered OPH degradation of nerve agent analog: paraoxon

2.1 Methods

2.1.1 Identify OPH mutation sites with molecular simulation

Computational studies, to identify OPH mutation sites, used chain A of the OPH crystal structure of paraoxon analog and diethyl 4-methylbenzylphosphonate, co-crystallized with OPH [5]. In contrast to most previous structural studies, which assumed that the binding orientation of paraoxon resembles the substrate analog [6–8], we identified a different binding mode for paraoxon compared to its analog diethyl 4-methylbenzylphosphonate [9]. To do this, we used three different docking algorithms (POSIT, HYBRID, and FRED) available in OPENEYE software

(OEDocking 3.2.0, OpenEye Inc.) to generate fifty potential binding modes of paraoxon in the OPH binding site. After down-selecting to the two most dissimilar paraoxon-OPH docking poses, we carried out molecular dynamics (MD) simulations over long times, up to 105 ns, to obtain the most stable paraoxon binding mode and define binding interactions at the OPH active site. MD simulation was also performed to identify mutation sites that can stabilize paraoxon binding.

Details of the MD simulations can be found in Ref. [9]. In brief, we used the OpenMM simulation package 7.11. We assigned partial charges to the substrate (paraoxon) atoms using the AM1-BCC charge model [10]. Amberff14SB and GAFF vs. 1.8 force fields were applied to the protein and substrate, respectively. We applied the TIP3P force field to describe water. After solvating the protein-substrate complex in water in a cubic box of 10 Å on a side, Na^+ and Cl^- counter ions were added to neutralize the system. We set the simulation time step to 4 fs and applied the hydrogen mass repartitioning approach [11, 12]. Long-ranged electrostatic interactions were calculated using the particle mesh Ewald approach [13], with a cut-off of 10 Å for the real-space electrostatic and Lennard-Jones forces. After minimizing the energy of the water and ions, while keeping the protein and substrate restrained using 500 kcal/mol-$Å^2$ positional restraints, we performed a second energy minimization step.

2.1.2 Cell-free protein synthesis of OPH variants

The rapid cell-free protein expression system can screen hundreds of variants per day in 200 μl reactions. The activity of the expressed product and substrate binding affinity also can be measured directly in the expression mixture, eliminating time-consuming and labor-intensive cell culture-based protein expression and purification processes. A wheat germ cell-free protein synthesis system from Cell-Free Science was used to generate wild type (WT) and mutant OPH. WT and mutant OPH plasmids were cloned into a pEU-E01 vector. The cell-free expression reaction is detailed here: 20 μl of transcription reactions containing 4 μl of 5x transcription buffer, 2 μl of NTP mix, 0.25 μl of RNase inhibitor, 0.25 μl of SP6 RNA polymerase, and 2 μl of plasmid are prepared and incubated at 37°C for 6 h, and then, translation reactions containing 10 μl of transcription reaction, 0.8 μl of creatine kinase (1 mg/ml), 10 μl of WEPRO, 75 μM of $Zn(OAc)_2$, and 206 μl of SUB-MIX are prepared and incubated at 15°C for 20 h. OPH variant expression in the cell-free reaction mixture was detected using SDS-gel. A series dilution of purified recombinant OPH was used as standards and loaded with cell-free generated OPH to a SDS gel, and OPH variant concentrations were determined by densitometry.

We also explored, for the first time, the possibility of using cell-free protein synthesis to express OPH with UAA substitutions. The small reaction volumes minimize the need for large quantities of UAAs. The plasmid encoding UAA tRNA/tRNA synthetase pair can be co-translated in the same cell-free reaction with expression protein; thus, the expensive and tricky re-engineering of living cellular expression systems is not required to accommodate a new genetic code for UAAs. In addition, the cell-free protein synthesis system's open access to transcription and translation simplifies protein expression optimization. To increase the chance of success, both wheat-germ and PURExpress cell-free system were used in this study. Six OPH mutants containing the amber codon for UAA substitution were constructed into both the PURExpress vector and pEU-E01 vector. Pilots of expression screening were performed with either co-translation of pAcFRS plasmid with OPH mutant plasmids in the same cell-free reaction or substitute reaction with pAcFRs protein and tRNA.

Ten UAAs were screened at various reaction conditions, including 4-acetyl-L-phenylalanine, 3,4 dihydroxy-L-phenylalanine, 1-methyl-L-histine, 4-amino-L-phenylalanine, 4,4,4,4,4,4-hexafluoro-valine, p-fluoro-phenylalanine, 5,5,5-trifluoro-leucine, 3,3,3-trifluoro-alanine, 1–4-thiazolylalanine, and L-3-thienylalanine. Only 4-acetyl-L-phenylalanine showed some level of expression in both cell-free systems, but kinetic measurement did not detect any activity on this UAA substitution. This expression was not confirmed beyond visual observation of a SDS gel band since this substitution was not active kinetically. More work can be done in the future by researchers who desire to advance the cell-free protein expression capability.

2.1.3 OPH UAA variant expression in cell culture

Eight OPH mutants containing an amber codon for UAA substitution were generated by GenScript. OPH-H55TAG, H57TAG, H201TAG, H230TAG, H254TAG, H257TAG, D253TAG, and D253E/H254TAG were cloned into pET24b(+) vector using NdeI/XhoI sites for expression in an *E. coli* host. The WT and mutant OPH cloned into pET24b(+) vector were co-transformed into the *E. coli* strain BL21 ai with proper GCE plasmids (**Table 1**). WT-GFP and GFP-150 plasmids were used as positive controls for UAA substitution. The cells were grown in standard LB supplemented with 1 mM UAA and induced by 0.2% L-arabinose and 1 mM IPTG at 16°C overnight. Cells were harvested by centrifugation at 4500 g for 15 min and resuspended in Ni-NTA lysis buffer: 50 mM NaH2PO4, 300 mM NaCl, 10 mM imidazole, and 0.1 μM pepstatin at a pH of 7.4. The cells were lysed using Microfluidizer (Microfluidics Corp, Westwood, MA) and then centrifuged at 12,000 g for 30 min. The collected supernatant was incubated with 5 ml of Ni-NTA resin under end-to-end shaking and loaded on a 5 mL HisTrap FF column. After washing with wash buffer containing 50 mM NaH_2PO_4, 300 mM NaCl, 20 mM imidazole, the proteins were eluted by elution

Mutant plasmid	Antibiotic resistance	GCE plasmid	Antibiotic resistance	UAA
H257TAG	Kanamycin (Kan)	pDulo-halo	Spectinomycin (Spec)	3,4-Dihydroxy-L-phenylalanine
H257TAG	Kan	pDulo-halo	Spec	3-BromoTyrosine
H257TAG	Kan	pDulo-pAminoPhe	Spec	4-Amino-L-phenylalanine
H55TAG	Kan	pEvol-pylRS-mjH	Chloramphenicol (Chl)	3-Methyl-Histine
H57TAG	Kan	pEvol-pylRS-mjH	Chl	3-Methyl-Histine
H201TAG	Kan	pEvol-pylRS-mjH	Chl	3-Methyl-Histine
H230TAG	Kan	pEvol-pylRS-mjH	Chl	3-Methyl-Histine
H254TAG	Kan	pEvol-pylRS-mjH	Chl	3-Methyl-Histine
H257TAG	Kan	pEvol-pylRS-mjH	Chl	3-Methyl-Histine
D253TAG	Kan	pEvol-pylRS-mjH	Chl	3-Methyl-Histine
D253E/H254TAG	Kan	pEvol-pylRS-mjH	Chl	3-Methyl-Histine

Table 1.
GCE plasmid and UAA combination used for co-transformation.

buffer containing 50 mM NaH_2PO_4, 300 mM NaCl, 250 mM imidazole. Elution fractions containing OPH UAA variants were pooled together and concentrated using a protein concentrator from Thermo Scientific.

2.1.4 Spectrophotometric assay of OPH variant activity

For cell-free synthesized OPH variants, their activities and substrate binding affinities were measured directly in the cell-free reaction mixture using a BioTek plate reader (Winooski, VT) and that reported light absorbance of the paraoxon leaving group at 405 nm. The assay conditions for cell-free expression were carried out by adding various amounts of paraoxon (final concentration: 0.1, 0.2, 0.5, 1.0, 2.0 and 3.0 mM) to 193.7 μL of buffer containing 100 mM CHES and 75 μM of $Zn(OAc)_2$, at pH = 9.0. The reactions were started by adding 2 μL of cell-free generated WT or OPH variants.

The kinetic assays of OPH UAA variants were performed also by measuring the absorbance of the paraoxon leaving group at 405 nm, as mentioned above. The changes of absorbance at 405 nm over time were used to calculate initial catalytic velocities as a function of the various substrate concentrations. Then, the initial velocity data, along with corresponding paraoxon concentrations, were plotted and analyzed by the Michaelis-Menten equation to obtain V_{max} and K_m using GraphPad (GraphPad Software, Inc., La Jolla, CA, USA). The k_{cat} was calculated by the ratio of V_{max} and mutant concentration. Each kinetic measurement condition was performed in triplicate and standard deviation was calculated using GraphPad.

2.2 Results

2.2.1 Identify OPH UAA mutation sites with increased active site stability

OPH used in this study is a homodimer from *Pseudomonas diminuta*. The OPH crystal structure 1HZY [1] contains 330 amino acids and two Zn(II) metal cations in Chain A. One Zn(II) coordinates with active site residues H201, H230 and two water molecules. The other Zn(II) coordinates with active site residues H55, H57, D301 and one water molecule [9]. Though OPH's natural substrate and function remains unknown, it is very effective at hydrolyzing the P—O bond of the phosphotriester insecticide paraoxon. OPH can also hydrolyze a wide spectrum of OP compounds containing phosphotriester (P—O), phosphonothioate (P—S), phosphonofluoridate (P—F), and phosphonocyanate (P—CN) bonds [14, 15].

Many previous studies on OPH focused only on altering the active site residues to achieve catalytic efficiency and substrate specificity. In this chapter, we extended our study of the OPH active site to include nearby active site residues as well, using the novel allosteric regulation approach. We targeted the residues near OPH active sites that do not coordinate with metal cations and are not involved in the hydrolysis reaction, but can form H-bonds with active site residues. In that way, we identified D253, which forms an H-bond with H230. An interesting observation about OPH is that its active site is dominated by four histidine residues: H55, H57, H201, and H230 (**Figure 1**). H254 and H257 also form an aromatic stacking network at the active site, while H257 plays an important role in stabilizing OPH [16]. We found that histidine's aromatic structure made it a great candidate for aromatic UAA substitution. Alterations of these histidine residues with UAA were achieved for examination of a more stable substrate binding reaction.

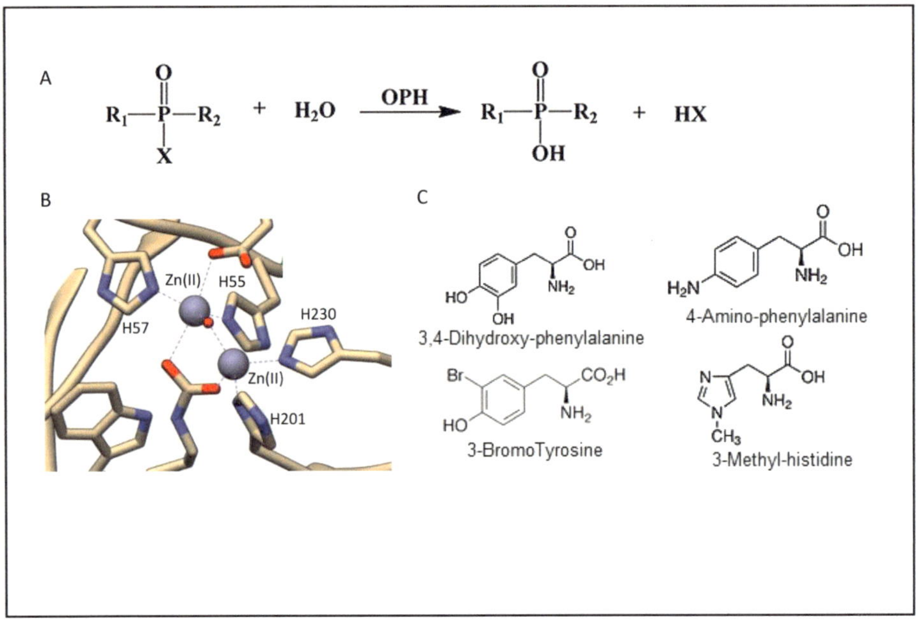

Figure 1.
A. Schematic diagram of OPH catalyzed hydrolysis reaction. B. OPH active site showing all four histidine residues and their interaction with Zn(II). C. Structure of UAAs used in this study.

2.2.2 Cell-free protein synthesis of OPH variants with increased thermal stability and substrate binding affinity

Despite the high-throughput advantage, a big challenge for many researchers has been how to maintain kinetic activity of expressed protein in cell-free protein synthesis system. Through screening of the cell-free reaction conditions, we have determined that the amount of creatine kinase played a key role in the success of OPH variant expression. Creatine kinase concentration was optimized and a large number of OPH variants were generated successfully using the cell-free protein synthesis system. Kinetic measurements were performed directly using the cell-free reaction mixture. Results of single mutation at D253E and double mutations at D253E/H254R both have improved paraoxon binding. Detailed study on OPH structure and kinetics on these two variants are reported in our recent publication [9]. In a separate study, we were interested in two threonine residues at allosteric location 54 and 199. We have examined the potential to replace threonine with a larger amino acid isoleucine to fill in the gap in OPH structure, therefore, to achieve active site stabilization. Single mutation at T199I and double mutation at T199I/T54I were not able to improve paraoxon binding affinity, but both mutations increased OPH kinetic activity up to 200-fold compared to WT OPH at temperature up to 60°C (manuscript under preparation), which shined light on OP agent remediation that requires OPH to function at elevated temperatures.

2.2.3 OPH UAA mutant expression in E. coli host

UAA substitution at H257 site was selected as an example to show expression level over time. The 4-amino-L-phenylalanine, 3,4-dihydroxy-L-phenylalanine, and

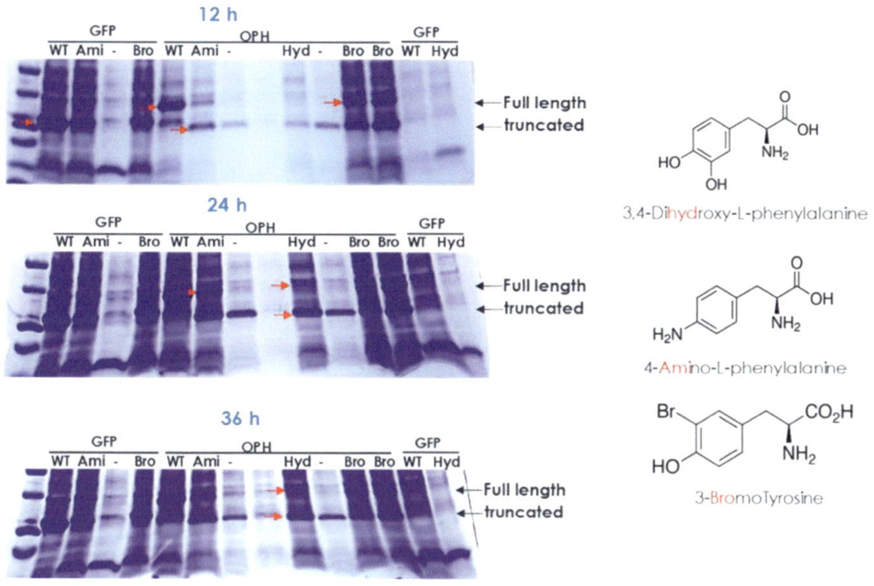

Figure 2.
Time course of OPH UAA substitution expression. Three UAAs were tested for expression over a time period of 36 h. GFP plasmids were used as positive control. UAA expression was detected starting at 12 h, and maintained up to 36 h. Letter abbreviations of UAA's full names are colored in red and to label UAA expression on SDS gels.

3-bromotyrosine substitutions at H257 were successfully expressed (**Figure 2**) over a 36-hour time period. Both 4-amino-L-phenylalanine and 3-bromotyrosine substitutions expressed at a relatively earlier time around 12 h, followed by 3,4-dihydroxy-L-phenylalanine substitution expression starting around 24 h. All substitutions are consistently expressed up to 36 h. The 3-methyl-histine substitution was also successfully expressed at H55, H57, H201, H230, H254, and H257. The 3-methyl-histine mutant expression level was higher than other three UAA substitutions due to close structural similarity to histidine.

2.2.4 Spectrophotometric assay of OPH UAA variant activity

The catalysis of P-O bond cleavage of paraoxon was monitored using a continuous spectrophotometric assay. Both k_{cat} and K_m values were measured and compared to WT OPH (**Table 2**). The 3,4-dihydroxy-L-phenylalanine substitution at H257 did not have any detectable activity. 4-amino-L-phenylalanine and 3-bromotyrosine substitutions at H257 resulted in a K_m of 0.018 mM and 0.073 mM, respectively (**Table 2**). The 4-amino-L-phenylalanine substitution at H257 improved paraoxon binding by 4.6-fold compared to WT OPH, while 3-bromo-tyrosine substitution at H257 did not improve paraoxon binding compared to WT OPH. Catalytic rates, k_{cat}, for these

	k_{cat} (s^{-1})	K_m (mM)	K_m fold improvement
WT OPH	25750.0 ± 2060.6	0.0835 ± 0.0186	—
H257-AminoPhe	—	0.0180 ± 0.0062	4.6
H257-BromoTyr	—	0.0728 ± 0.0146	1.1
H257-HydroxyPhe	—	—	—
H55-MethylHis	588.9 ± 27.3	0.0265 ± 0.0055	3.2
H57-MethylHis	221.0 ± 24.2	0.2346 ± 0.0719	0.36
H201-MethylHis	2.5 ± 0.1	0.0174 ± 0.0024	4.8
H230-MethylHis	4.9 ± 0.1	0.0058 ± 0.0005	14.4
H254-MethylHis	25.6 ± 0.9	0.0254 ± 0.0046	3.3
H257-MethylHis	56.0 ± 3.0	0.0459 ± 0.0096	1.8
D253-MethylHis	2.0 ± 0.2	0.2137 ± 0.0660	0.4
D253E-H254MethylHis	2.6 ± 0.3	0.0991 ± 0.0318	0.8

Table 2.
The k_{cat} and K_m measured for WT and mutant OPH.

mutants were not calculated due to low protein concentration after elution from Ni-NTA column, which made protein concentration measurement impossible.

Non-histidine residue UAA substitution at D253 was not able to improve substrate binding. This aligns with our hypothesis that our selected UAAs are more suitable for histidine replacement.

All 3-methyl-histine substitutions are kinetically active (**Table 2**). The 3-methyl-histine substitution at H230 resulted in the most improvement among all mutants, with a 14.4-fold increase in paraoxon binding. The 3-methyl-histine substitution at H55 was the most active mutant, with a 3.2-fold increase in paraoxon binding.

2.3 Discussion

An effective enzyme bio-engineering approach starts by the identification of key amino acid residues that, when altered, improve the activity of the targeted enzyme. Many successes have been demonstrated through the development of small molecule binding proteins [17] and redesign of enzyme binding sites to either accommodate a new substrate [18] or engineer novel catalytic sites [19, 20]. A few promising results in developing potential therapeutics have examined the applications of allosteric regulations in protein engineering [21–30].

OPH is capable of hydrolyzing a wide spectrum of OP compounds, but its application in neurotoxin degradation was limited due to insufficient substrate binding affinity. In our previous project on developing thermally stable OPH variants, we utilized an allosteric network modulation algorithm and molecular design suite "Eris" [31, 32]. Hotspots that enhanced allosteric network stability were identified and we produced dozens of OPH mutants exhibiting enhanced kinetics for paraoxon, but none of them improved substrate binding. Saturation mutagenesis done by Chen et al. also failed to tighten substrate binding [33].

In this work, we investigated the potential of using UAA substitutions to improve OPH substrate binding. OPH has a unique active site structure packed with histidine residues. These histidine residues form aromatic stacking network and H-bond with substrate. Three GCE plasmids and four UAAs were tested successfully for OPH UAA expression. Among four UAA substitutions, 3,4-dihydroxy-L-phenylalanine substitution not only needed longer time to express, but also resulted in no detectable activity. The 3-bromotyrosine substitutions expressed well, with low yield after purification, but this substitution was not able to improve substrate binding. These observations eliminate both compounds from the potential UAA substitution list. The 4-amino-L-phenylalanine substitution expressed well, with a low protein yield after purification. This result makes kinetic measurement difficult. With a 4.6-fold improvement on substrate binding, further optimization on protein expression could still make 4-amino-L-phenylalanine a good UAA substitution candidate. The 3-methyl-His replacement achieved the highest protein expression level, and the 3-methyl-His replacement at H230 expressed the highest improvement on paraoxon binding. 3-methyl-His replacement at H230 was able to bring K_m down to 5.8 μM, close to the nerve agent lethal dose. Since H230 is located at the OPH active site, the 3-methyl-His replacement also reduced the turnover rate of this mutation. Force fields for these UAAs are not currently available, so MD simulation cannot yet be used to examine UAA orientations at the active site nor any formation of H-bond after UAA substitution. The goal of this study is to demonstrate the proof-of-concept of the feasibility of using UAA substitution to stabilize the OPH active site and improve substrate binding affinity. Our results are promising and provide new insight into OPH bioengineering.

2.4 Conclusion

In this chapter, we demonstrated the high-throughput of cell-free protein synthesis in enzyme kinetic studies. We also explored the possibility of using UAA to enhance OPH substrate binding by testing a method utilizing GCE machinery to incorporate selected UAAs into OPH. A TAG stop codon was inserted into OPH to replace these sites, and OPH mutants with UAA substitution were expressed successfully. A total of eleven UAA substitutions were generated, with 3-methyl-histine substitutions identified as the most suitable to replace the OPH active site histidine network. Results of kinetic studies of these mutants show significantly improved OPH substrate binding affinity.

Acknowledgements

The team would like to thank Sandia's LDRD program.

Sandia National Laboratories (SNL) is a multi-mission laboratory managed and operated by National Technology & Engineering Solutions of Sandia, LLC, a wholly owned subsidiary of Honeywell International Inc., for the U.S. Department of Energy's National Nuclear Security Administration under contract DE-NA0003525. This work was supported by Sandia's LDRD program. The views expressed in the article do not necessarily represent the views of the U.S. Department of Energy or the United States Government.

Author details

Dongmei Ye* and Susan Rempe
Sandia National Laboratories, Albuquerque, New Mexico, USA

*Address all correspondence to: dye@sandia.gov

References

[1] Talabani JM, Ali AI, Kadir AM, Rashid R, Samin F, Greenwood D, et al. Long-term health effects of chemical warfare agents on children following a single heavy exposure. Human & Experimental Toxicology. 2018;**37**:836-847

[2] Smart JK, editor. History of Chemical and Biological Warfare: An American Perspective. Falls Church, Virginia: Office of The Surgeon General, Department of the Army; 2008. pp. 9-76

[3] Kim M, Gkikas M, Huang A, Kang JW, Suthiwangcharoen N, Nagarajan R, et al. Enhanced activity and stability of organophosphorus hydrolase via interaction with an amphiphilic polymer. Chemical Communication (Camb). 2014;**50**:5345-5348

[4] Otto TC, Harsch CK, Yeung DT, Magliery TJ, Cerasoli DM, Lenz DE. Dramatic differences in organophosphorus hydrolase activity between human and chimeric recombinant mammalian paraoxonase-1 enzymes. Biochemistry. 2009;**48**:10416-10422

[5] Benning MM, Shim H, Raushel FM, Holden HM. High resolution X-ray structures of different metal-substituted forms of phosphotriesterase from Pseudomonas diminuta. Biochemistry. 2001;**40**:2712-2722

[6] Wong KY, Gao J. The reaction mechanism of paraoxon hydrolysis by phosphotriesterase from combined QM/MM simulations. Biochemistry. 2007;**46**:13352-13369

[7] Koca J, Zhan CG, Rittenhouse RC, Ornstein RL. Mobility of the active site bound paraoxon and sarin in zinc-phosphotriesterase by molecular dynamics simulation and quantum chemical calculation. Journal of the American Chemical Society. 2001;**123**:817-826

[8] Gomes DE, Lins RD, Pascutti PG, Lei C, Soares TA. Conformational variability of organophosphorus hydrolase upon soman and paraoxon binding. The Journal of Physical Chemistry. B. 2011;**115**:15389-15398

[9] El Khoury L, Mobley DL, Ye D, Rempe SB. Enhancing Paraoxon binding to organophosphorus hydrolase active site. International Journal of Molecular Sciences. 2021;**22**:12624-12640

[10] Hopkins CW, Le Grand S, Walker RC, Roitberg AE. Long-time-step molecular dynamics through hydrogen mass repartitioning. Journal of Chemical Theory and Computation. 2015;**11**:1864-1874

[11] Darden TY, Pedersen L. Particle mesh Ewald: An N log (N) method for Ewald sums in large systems. The Journal of Chemical Physics. 1993;**98**:10089-10092

[12] Onufriev A, Bashford D, Case DA. Exploring protein native states and large-scale conformational changes with a modified generalized born model. Proteins. 2004;**55**:383-394

[13] Axelsen PHL. Improved convergence in dual-topology free energy calculations through use of harmonic restraints. Journal of Computational Chemistry. 1998;**19**:1278-1283

[14] Lewis VE, Donarski WJ, Wild JR, Raushel FM. Mechanism and stereochemical course at phosphorus of the reaction catalyzed by a bacterial phosphotriesterase. Biochemistry. 1988;**27**:1591-1597

[15] Aubert SD, Li Y, Raushel FM. Mechanism for the hydrolysis of organophosphates by the bacterial phosphotriesterase. Biochemistry. 2004;**43**:5707-5715

[16] Reeves TE, Wales ME, Grimsley JK, Li P, Cerasoli DM, Wild JR. Balancing the stability and the catalytic specificities of OP hydrolases with enhanced V-agent activities. Protein Engineering, Design & Selection. 2008;**21**:405-412

[17] Tinberg CE, Khare SD, Dou J, Doyle L, Nelson JW, Schena A, et al. Computational design of ligand-binding proteins with high affinity and selectivity. Nature. 2013;**501**:212-216

[18] Grisewood MJ, Gifford NP, Pantazes RJ, Li Y, Cirino PC, Janik MJ, et al. OptZyme: Computational enzyme redesign using transition state analogues. PLoS One. 2013;**8**:e75358

[19] Bjelic S, Kipnis Y, Wang L, Pianowski Z, Vorobiev S, Su M, et al. Exploration of alternate catalytic mechanisms and optimization strategies for retroaldolase design. Journal of Molecular Biology. 2014;**426**:256-271

[20] Rajagopalan S, Wang C, Yu K, Kuzin AP, Richter F, Lew S, et al. Design of activated serine-containing catalytic triads with atomic-level accuracy. Nature Chemical Biology. 2014;**10**:386-391

[21] Wild C, Cunningham KA, Zhou J. Allosteric modulation of G protein-coupled receptors: An emerging approach of drug discovery. Austin Journal of Pharmacological Therapy. 2014;**2014**:2

[22] De Smet F, Christopoulos A, Carmeliet P. Allosteric targeting of receptor tyrosine kinases. Nature Biotechnology. 2014;**32**:1113-1120

[23] Nickols HH, Conn PJ. Development of allosteric modulators of GPCRs for treatment of CNS disorders. Neurobiology of Disease. 2014;**61**:55-71

[24] Wang L, Martin B, Brenneman R, Luttrell LM, Maudsley S. Allosteric modulators of g protein-coupled receptors: Future therapeutics for complex physiological disorders. The Journal of Pharmacology and Experimental Therapeutics. 2009;**331**:340-348

[25] Karginov AV, Ding F, Kota P, Dokholyan NV, Hahn KM. Engineered allosteric activation of kinases in living cells. Nature Biotechnology. 2010;**28**:743-747

[26] Wenthur CJ, Gentry PR, Mathews TP, Lindsley CW. Drugs for allosteric sites on receptors. Annual Review of Pharmacology and Toxicology. 2014;**54**:165-184

[27] Wootten D, Christopoulos A, Sexton PM. Emerging paradigms in GPCR allostery: Implications for drug discovery. Nature Reviews. Drug Discovery. 2013;**12**:630-644

[28] Dokholyan NV. Controlling allosteric networks in proteins. Chemical Reviews. 2016;**116**:6463-6487

[29] Dagliyan O, Tarnawski M, Chu PH, Shirvanyants D, Schlichting I, Dokholyan NV, et al. Engineering extrinsic disorder to control protein activity in living cells. Science. 2016;**354**:1441-1444

[30] Dagliyan O, Shirvanyants D, Karginov AV, Ding F, Fee L, Chandrasekaran SN, et al. Rational design of a ligand-controlled protein conformational switch. Proceedings of the National Academy of Sciences of the United States of America. 2013;**110**:6800-6804

[31] Yin S, Ding F, Dokholyan NV. Modeling backbone flexibility improves protein stability estimation. Structure. 2007;**15**:1567-1576

[32] Yin S, Ding F, Dokholyan NV. Eris: An automated estimator of protein stability. Nature Methods. 2007;**4**:466-467

[33] Mee-Hie Cho C, Mulchandani A, Chen W. Functional analysis of organophosphorus hydrolase variants with high degradation activity towards organophosphate pesticides. Protein Engineering, Design & Selection. 2006;**19**:99-105